Diagnostic Microbiology and Cytology of the Eye

Diagnostic Microbiology and Cytology of the Eye

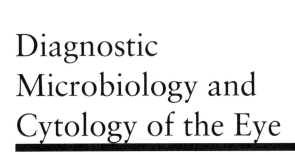
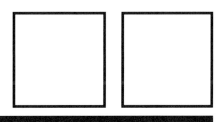

KATHLEEN A. BYRNE, M.T.

Research Associate and Microbiologist
Department of Ophthalmology
College of Medicine
King Saud University
Riyadh, Saudi Arabia
and Ocular Microbiologist
Poulsbo, Washington

EILEEN M. BURD, Ph.D.

Department of Ophthalmology
The Eye Institute
Medical College of Wisconsin
Milwaukee, Wisconsin

KHALID F. TABBARA, M.D.

Professor and Chairman
Department of Ophthalmology
College of Medicine
King Saud University
Riyadh, Saudi Arabia

ROBERT A. HYNDIUK, M.D.

Professor of Ophthalmology
The Eye Institute
Medical College of Wisconsin
Milwaukee, Wisconsin

Foreword by: Chandler R. Dawson, M.D., Director of the Proctor Foundation, San Francisco, California

Butterworth–Heinemann

Boston • Oxford • Melbourne • Singapore • Toronto • Munich • New Delhi • Tokyo

Every effort has been made to ensure that the drug dosage schedules within this text are accurate
and conform to standards accepted at time of publication. However, as treatment recommendations vary in the light of continuing research and clinical experience, the reader is advised to ver-
ify drug dosage schedules herein with information found on product information sheets. This is
especially true in cases of new or infrequently used drugs.

∞ Recognizing the importance of preserving what has been written, it is the policy of Butterworth–Heinemann to have the books it publishes printed on acid-free paper, and we exert our
best efforts to that end.

Library of Congress Cataloging-in-Publication Data

Diagnostic microbiology and cytology of the eye / Kathleen A. Byrne
   . . . [et al.] ; foreword by director of the Proctor Institute.
       p.   cm.
   Includes bibliographical references and index.
   ISBN 0-7506-9607-9 (acid-free paper)
     1. Eye—Infections—Diagnosis. 2. Eye—Infections—Cytodiagnosis.
I. Byrne, Kathleen A.
RE96.D52 1995
617.7'1—dc20   94-28598
                                                                CIP

British Library Cataloging-in-Publication Data

A catalog record for this book is available from the British Library.

Butterworth–Heinemann
313 Washington Street
Newton, MA 02158-1626

10   9   8   7   6   5   4   3   2   1

Printed in the United States of America

To our mentor and teacher Dr. Phillips Thygeson, Professor Emeritus, University of California, San Francisco, California. Dr. Thygeson is the pioneer and father of modern ocular microbiology and cytology.

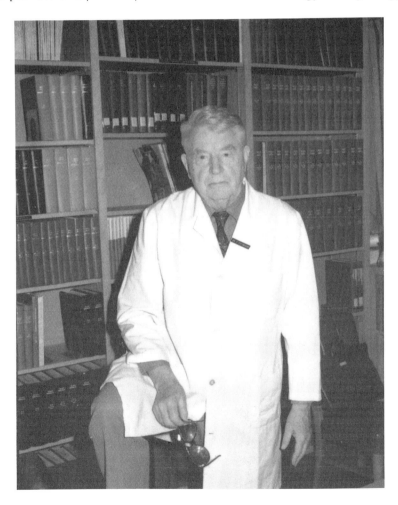

Contents

Preface

Although many comprehensive procedure manuals exist in clinical microbiology, there remains a need for a manual that guides us in the multidisciplinary practices of methods in ocular microbiology and the cytology of cellular immune responses. There are a number of tests involved in characterizing and identifying the causative agent in infectious diseases of the eye that may exhaust the resources and capabilities of many clinical laboratories. Therefore we have extracted from journals, textbooks in clinical microbiology, and reference manuals, as well as the authors' personal experiences, to provide a collection of techniques and alternative procedures most useful in the definitive diagnosis of ocular pathogens and indigenous flora. Microbiologists are often consulted concerning the types of specimens required for microscopy, culture examination, and studies of unusual pathogens; so care has been taken to include eye scrapings and procedures that may be performed by clinicians or other health care personnel. The authors wish to thank Luis E. Barrantes, owner of Poulsbo 1-Hour Photographic Studios in Washington State and husband of K. Byrne, for his technical advice and professional photographic work in the preparation of the slides and color plates contained in this manual. We also would like to state our appreciation to the people who provided some of the slides as a courtesy to the production of this work, whom we have given credit in the legend. These scientists and those mentioned in the following referenced work have contributed much to the field of research and laboratory medicine. And a word of thanks to David Bray III, M.D., Pathologist, Washington State, for his review of the histopathologic slides and input from the standpoint of a clinical laboratory in a rural setting. We also acknowledge the support of Mr. Abdul-Rahman Saad Al-Rashed Fund for Research in Ophthalmology. We hope that this work will find its way to the shelves of many clinical, research, and pathology laboratories, and ophthalmologist's practices; we have tried to incorporate everything from the first step in the front office to the final result and therapeutic monitoring of ocular microbiologic and cytologic investigations.

Ocular Microbiology and Cytology: Purpose

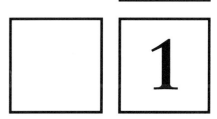

Medicine has become a wide variety of disciplines with many subspecialities. Clinical microbiologists play an important role in the diagnosis and management of many preventable and curable ocular disorders. Ocular microbiology and cytology are two areas that have seen major advances in past decades.

1.1. PURPOSE OF DIAGNOSTIC OCULAR MICROBIOLOGY

The role of the clinical microbiologist is to work closely with ophthalmologists, clinicians, and other members of the health care team to provide diagnosis and expeditious management of infectious eye disease and to take precautions to prevent the spread of these infections to others. This is undertaken by the careful and accurate handling of cultures and patients, the determination of the cause of the illness, and the proper documentation of these findings. In many cases of infectious disease there may be little time to save the eye. Ocular infections may progress to cerebrospinal and brain involvement, septicemia, and death. Therefore, early diagnosis and treatment of ocular infections are more urgent than in many other types of disease processes, and loss of sight or even death can be significantly reduced when guided by the knowledge of the causative organism, cytologic changes, and results of antimicrobial susceptibility testing. Accurate and responsible record keeping, specimen collection, setup and handling of culture results, proper quality control, understanding of microbes common in ocular infections, recovery of causative organisms, and specific identification and antimicrobial testing are critical to a favorable outcome in the case of eye disease. A differential diagnosis may be based initially on the

1

clinical picture or on results of ultrasound, radiology, blood tests, and other ophthalmic evaluations. It is the expertise of the competent microbiologist in interpreting tests and the ophthalmologist's astute discernment of the most useful laboratory analyses for definitive diagnosis that allows the health care team to perform with maximum efficiency.

1.2. PURPOSE OF OCULAR CYTOLOGY AND CELLULAR IMMUNE RESPONSES

The examination of cells from cornea and conjunctival scrapings or exudates may provide invaluable information in making or substantiating the diagnosis in infectious disease of the eye. The presence or predominance of certain types of inflammatory cells or changes in the epithelial cells often indicate a specific disease state. The absence or reduced number of certain others, such as goblet cells, may indicate dry eye states, including vitamin A deficiency, and may be useful in monitoring the efficacy of treatment in dry eye disorders. Recognizing keratinization and other neoplastic processes such as nuclear enlargement or multinucleation may be an indication of ocular tumors or infection of *Chlamydia trachomatis.* Viral intranuclear or chlamydial intracytoplasmic inclusion bodies may be present within the epithelial cell and are visible in a well-stained smear. In addition to the identification of peripheral blood cells that may be found in an eye scraping, the microbiologist/cytologist must be able to recognize certain early cells such as blast cells, plasma cells, mast cells, and a type of macrophage unique to the eye referred to as "Leber cells," which were named after the ophthalmologist who first described them. Macrophages may be found in certain types of conjunctivitis, herpesvirus infections, and in phacoanaphylactic endophthalmitis; engulfing lens and iral pigment as seen in Plate 1. The morphology, stain characteristics, appropriate types of stain, alternate tests, as well as the clinical significance of ocular cytology are detailed in the following chapters. Color plates of stained smears and clinical pictures as well as referenced supplemental readings are provided, which may aid in establishing a diagnosis of common and unusual disease processes. Other findings, such as parasitic infestation of amoebic keratitis, microsporidiosis, malarial parasites, or *Malassezia furfur* yeast (Plate 2), which do not turn up by standard culture techniques, may first be found using cytologic stains such as Giemsa, Hematoxylin & Eosin, Papanicolaou, Grocott-Gomori methenamine silver, Calcofluor white, and others. The indication for use of special stains and the most useful combination of these to establish definitive diagnoses based on suspected pathogens are included when pertinent. Special tests, reagents, fixatives, and other recommendations useful within the microbiology laboratory or referral laboratories are explained by following these procedures from specimen collection to stains to culture to antibiotics to expected results and quality control.

1.3. NONCULTURAL METHODS OF DIAGNOSIS

The clinician depends on data from many sources in arriving at tentative or definitive diagnosis. Technical advances in laboratory procedures and instrumentation such as electron microscopy, monoclonal antibodies, genetic probes, gas liquid chromatography for demonstration of volatile metabolic end products, enzyme-linked immunoassay, polymerase chain reaction techniques in molecular biology, certain skin tests, and serologic evaluation of immune responses are all useful in the differential diagnosis of ocular infections and neoplasias. Often it is necessary to include a combination of these rather than to depend exclusively on just one. Because this is a microbiology and cytology procedure manual, those procedures that may be performed within the microbiology sections are detailed but, when possible and important, comparison studies and alternate tests are suggested within the scope of laboratory medicine. It is hoped that although the testing may be done outside the microbiology laboratory, the microbiologist and ophthalmologist might be aware of the significance of these results in interpreting the workup within the microbiology and cytology sections. Further findings and supplemental readings are provided in referenced text as they relate to a specific suspected organism or disease process.

Clerical Procedures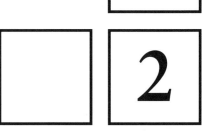

It is important that a system be set up in the clinical laboratory for the proper handling and processing of ocular specimens and that criteria for specimen collection and transportation be efficient and provide means of documentation of time of receipt and specimen acceptability. The quality of a laboratory's work is contingent on the timely receipt of a specimen and its condition on arrival to the microbiology and pathology laboratories. Accurate record keeping and detailed patient information may be crucial in the interpretation and workup of the entire culture or of histologic studies. Therefore, a consistent procedure for record keeping, computer entries in patient files, specimen reception, and labeling is an important part of this process. Because computer systems and clerical procedures vary widely among institutions, the following is intended as a guide to what information is necessary and to establish a criteria for specimen rejection and special handling to yield favorable results.

2.1 RECEPTION DETAILS

Specimens are generally received from both inpatient and outpatient areas or clinics by the specimen reception area of the clinical laboratory, where they are verified with time of receipt and subsequently delivered to the appropriate laboratory or department. It is important to indicate the exact time and date the specimen was received in the laboratory. Specimens for processing by only Pathology, Electron Microscopy, or Research should be brought to these sections or laboratories directly because they may require special handling. Specimens that require processing in both clinical microbiology and other sections or laboratories should be processed for the microbiology procedures first to avoid contamination from nonsterile handling. After processing for the clinical procedures requested, they should be delivered as soon as possible to the respective laboratory.

2.2. LABORATORY REQUEST FORMS

All specimens brought to the clinical laboratory should be accompanied by a laboratory request form or computer-generated order and labeling system on which the following information should appear:

2.2.1. Patient Data

Patient's medical record number
Patient's name
Ward or outpatient area
Age/Sex
Nationality

2.2.2. Specimen Data

Source of specimen (i.e., conjunctiva, cornea, fluid)
Procedures requested (culture, Giemsa, special stains, or unusual pathogens suspected)
Date and time collected
Date and time specimen was received in the laboratory

2.2.3. Doctor Data

The name of the doctor ordering the test
Name of doctor requesting copy of results (if different from above)
Consulting doctor

This information is needed so that the physician may be informed of results and to facilitate communication when necessary.

2.2.4. Miscellaneous Data

Diagnosis and clinical impression
Antibiotic therapy
Patient's immune status (i.e., cancer therapy, HIV positive, transplant surgery, etc.)

Any other information that may help in interpretation of results or aid in the workup where special media or stains may be required.

2.2.5. Missing Information

If any information is missing or is not legible, it is necessary to find or call the doctor or hospital floor, then indicate the correct information on the laboratory slip or in the computer as soon as possible. If certain information is not available or the doctor is not available, let someone know (i.e., nurse taking care of patient or clinic assistant, etc.) that this information is necessary and request that the doctor or other health care individual call the laboratory as soon as possible.

2.3 ACCESSIONING OF SPECIMEN AND CRITERIA FOR ACCEPTABILITY

2.3.1. Accessioning of Specimens for Microbiologic Evaluation

A computer file or running log book should be maintained for all incoming specimens to the clinical laboratory, and this may sometimes include a flow sheet for specimens that will also be sent to other sections or laboratories. Information should include that listed in section 2.2 and a space for the date on which the final report is issued. Specimens and requisitions are then given an accession number. The number and sometimes additional information such as name, account or medical record number, and test ordered may be printed by computerized labeling systems already in use in the clinical laboratory. This number must appear on all copies of the requisitions, worksheets, plates, slides, tubes of inoculated media, including those that may be hand written during subsequent testing of positive cultures and smears requiring additional special stains.

2.3.2 Criteria for Acceptability of Specimens

Before plating or performing staining procedures, the specimen and the requisition form both must be examined for acceptability. This prevents unnecessary workup of poor-quality specimens and avoids labeling errors. An acceptable requisition should have complete information, as described in 2.2. The specimen container should be labeled with much of the same information, but must include minimum information such as the patient's full name, location or bed number, and the date and time at which the specimen was collected. Unlabeled specimens are not acceptable in a clinical laboratory. If the label is not complete or is incorrect, the nurse or clinician should be called to identify the specimen, and laboratory personnel should note this on the requisition and in an incident report book. This is of utmost importance because the subsequent workup of positives and treatment of patient may be adversely affected by a possible mix-up of specimens. The specimen must be in an appropriate container and must have correct transport medium for culture.

Specimens should be obtained so as to preclude or minimize the possibility of introducing extraneous microorganisms that may not be involved in the infectious process. The entire workup and cost to laboratory and patient may be affected by the reporting of a false-positive result. If the specimen is not appropriate in any way, a new specimen should be requested by telephone immediately. If a new specimen cannot be obtained, consult the ordering physician before processing the specimen. If several procedures are requested and there is not enough material to perform all, consult the patient's physician to determine a plan of action for working up the tests that will provide the most important information. This can sometimes be guided by the results of initial smears. This is where the microbiologist should not hesitate to communicate with the clinician on possible pathogens and techniques that may be useful in differential diagnosis. Frequently, it is necessary and important to do the best job possible on a small volume or a less-than-optimal specimen.

2.4. RESULT REPORTS

All results of smears, cultures, and sometimes of noncultural methods including serologies must be recorded in a Microbiology Log Book or released in the computer and maintained in a separate or ongoing positive file with the date the report was sent out. Some testing results are immediately finalized, on the same day, after the test is performed. Others may require preliminary and also interim reports during culture workups and lengthy incubation periods; this information is contained in later chapters. Generally, reports are sent out at 1 or 2 days, 7 days, and 2 weeks, with results of smears being reported as soon as possible or on the same day the specimen was received in the case of Gram and Giemsa stains.

2.4.1 Preliminary and Interim Reports

With most ocular cultures, and particularly with cornea and intraocular fluids, a 24-hour report is sent. Any change in culture status from the initial 24-hour report also should be released as soon as possible and sometimes called to the clinician, inpatient floor, or ward nurse in charge. An interim report is also indicated for those cultures with multiple isolates, which may cause a delay in sending out a final report.

2.4.2. Final Reports

All final reports are generally made in quadruplicate (for distribution) and initialed by the microbiologist or supervisor. In many computer systems the final release is generated by the supervisor or another microbiologist to eliminate possible clerical errors. The reports then are filed, with one copy to the doctor, one copy for medical records, one for billing, and a department copy.

2.5. STATISTICAL RECORDS

A final copy of the report should be maintained in a separate log or file within microbiology to ease retrieval and monitoring of antibiotic sensitivities and statistics. Most institutions also require a copy to be given to the Infection Control nurse and sometimes the pharmacy in the case of antibiotic sensitivities. Some of the information from these statistics is of value when requests for personnel, laboratory equipment, and laboratory space increases are made.

Setup Procedures and Specimen Collection Protocol

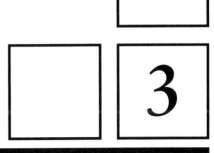

3

There have been major advances in the scope of the microbiologic investigation of ocular infections. The collection and safe management of clinical specimens in the laboratory is largely determined by the site of infection, severity of disease process, and likelihood of causative organisms. The quality of a laboratory's definitive diagnosis of a wide variety of possible pathogens is dependent on proper collection and expeditious handling of specimens, using appropriate culture media and stains for smears or other procedures. The microbiologist must be prepared to assist the clinician in choosing a rational approach through knowledge of the roles of various bacteria, viruses, and parasites in ocular disease processes. The ophthalmologist should become familiar with the various tests available in the laboratory and be willing to offer suggestions and communicate their needs to laboratory personnel in cases where unusual pathogens are suspected. Special procedures are required to collect and process the small quantity of material from the eye. Because of the small amount of material that can be obtained from an infected site in the eye and because both positive and negative results are used to make a diagnosis, the quality of the specimen is critical. Proper handling of specimens is equally critical because these specimens cannot usually be replaced by additional material. Certain stains require different fixatives, and bedside or direct culture in the clinic or hospital room offer a better chance of survival for many fastidious organisms that cause eye infections. The laboratory should ensure that the materials needed for specimen collection are available in the operating room, inpatient units, and affiliated outpatient units. The following procedures for setup of cultures and smears and protocol for direct inoculation serve as a guide to what may be necessary to retrieve and process specimens within the clinical or research laboratory.

Suggestions are given for working up small quantities and special handling of material for routine, fungal, mycobacterial, cell culture, parasitic investigation, histologic studies, electron microscopy, and currently recommended stains for accurate identification. Detailed descriptions for interpreting results of stained smears and complete culture workups are contained in the following chapters. The ideal selection of media can and should be modified according to individual circumstances and the scope of services offered in a particular laboratory. Because many specimens obtained from the eye are irreplaceable, it is important that proper protocols be firmly established and followed so that each specimen is handled to optimize recovery of pathogens. The ophthalmologists also may need to familiarize themselves with the availability of certain reference laboratories and universities that the local laboratory service may use so that specimens may be sent out for special tests. Many of these institutions offer courier services and special taxis to collect specimens from remote or rural areas.

3.1 SPECIMEN COLLECTION DEVICES

Kimura platinum spatula: for obtaining material from cornea and conjunctival scrapings. The platinum tip (Figure 3.1) may be heat sterilized between uses with a bactericidal incinerator or flame; it cools rapidly. Used for direct inoculation of culture plates and smears, broths, and viral or *Chlamydia* transport media

Sterile anaerobic and aerobic transport swabs: may be used for specimen collection and transport to laboratory while the specimen is being maintained

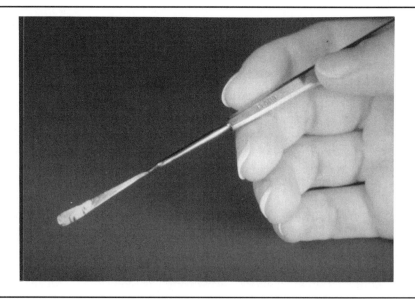

Figure 3.1
Platinum-tip Kimura spatula used for ocular scrapings.

in a support media. Many brands and systems are available, but these should never be used for smears because they introduce too many artifacts that may interfere with stain reaction and interpretations.

Needle and syringe: preferred method for collecting fluid or pus for routine and anaerobic cultures. May also be used to transport to laboratory, but the needle must be removed and disposed of in a biohazard container before transporting to the laboratory

Dacron, polyester, or rayon swabs: may be used to collect material for cell cultures. Scrapings are preferred, but swabs may be used to collect excess material after the pustule is opened or debridement is performed. Cotton, calcium alginate, and swabs with wooden shafts should never be used because they have been shown to affect certain isolates.

Frosted, etched, and cleaned glass slides with transport carrier: used for direct preparation of smears for staining. Note: Slides must be cleaned using methyl alcohol and air-dried because most slides, even precleaned brands, have a thin film coating that may cause organisms and cells to wash off during the staining process.

3.2. MEDIA REQUIRED FOR COLLECTION

Routine and special media (Figure 3.2) include the following:

Thioglycolate broth: used as a general all-purpose nutrient broth medium for both anaerobic and aerobic bacteria and useful for moistening swabs for specimen collection

Defibrinated sheep blood (5%) in a nutrient agar base: suitable for the growth of most bacteria and yeasts or fungi

Chocolate blood agar (peptone base, enriched with solution of 2% hemoglobin or chemical supplements such as IsovitaleX [BBL]): suitable for the growth of most bacteria but necessary for the cultivation of *Neisseria spp, Haemophilus spp,* and certain nutritionally variant species of *Streptococcus.*

Thayer Martin medium or New York City (NYC) agar (peptone or blood agar base with vitamin supplements and antibiotic supplements such as vancomycin, nystatin, etc. to inhibit the growth of contaminating organisms and yeast): Used for the selective isolation of *Neisseria gonorrhoeae* and *Neisseria meningitidis* suspected infections

Sabouraud's dextrose agar (Emmons modification): suitable for the isolation of most fungi, yeasts, Actinomycetes, and suspected *Nocardia spp.* Should also be set up on LJ or MB 7H10 or 7H11 slants described below

Lowenstein-Jensen (LJ) Egg-based medium (contaminants are inhibited by malachite green): for the primary isolation of mycobacteria such as *Mycobacterium tuberculosis* as well as a typical species (nontuberculous mycobacteria)

Nonnutritive agar to which a fresh suspension of *Escherichia coli* or *Klebsiella pneumoniae* in Page's amoeba saline is overlayed after inoculation (see reagents section): for suspected amoebic keratitis of *Acanthamoeba spp* or *Naegleria fowleri.*

Brain Heart Infusion Broth (BHI) or chopped meat broth: Recommended for the isolation of nutritive variant bacteria. Chopped meat has an increased

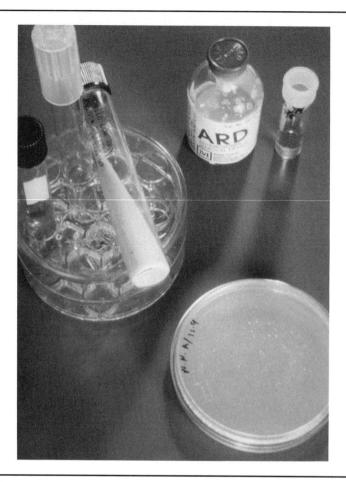

Figure 3.2
Broths and culture media such as Lowenstein-Jensen or nonnutrient agars that may be required for unusual pathogens and nutritional variants.

chance of bacterial recovery when antibiotics have been given because the chopped meat has been shown to absorb some of the chemicals. However, an antimicrobial removal device is recommended for this use if available.

Viral and/or *Chlamydia* transport media (some brands support both; however, please read manufacturer's instructions before use): used for viral and *Chlamydia trachomatis* cultures and, when refrigerated, will hold organisms viable before processing in cell culture for up to 3 days

BIBLIOGRAPHY

1. In Baron EJ, Peterson L, Finegold SM (eds): Cultivation and isolation of viable pathogens. Bailey and Scott's diagnostic microbiology. Chapter 9. 9th Edition. St. Louis: Mosby, 1994: 80–83.

2. Jones DB, Liesegang TJ, Robinson NM, Washington JA. Cumitech 13, laboratory diagnosis of ocular infections, cumulative techniques and procedures in clinical microbiology. Washington, DC: American Society of Microbiology, May 1981.
3. Mandell GL, Douglas RG, Bennett JE (eds): Principles and practices of infectious diseases. 3rd Edition. New York: Churchill Livingstone.1990.
4. Washington JA (ed): Laboratory procedures in clinical microbiology. New York: Springer-Verlag, 1981.

3.3 SPECIMEN COLLECTION PROTOCOLS

The following procedures should be performed by the clinician or ophthalmologist and others who may have special training to perform direct inoculation of culture media and slides at bedside or in the clinic or hospital areas. In cases of infectious keratitis, it is recommended that the lid and conjunctiva be cultured before performing a corneal debridement so as not to introduce any contaminants or normal flora of the ocular adnexa. These cultures are then useful in determining whether isolates from the corneal cultures could be normal flora from the lids and conjunctiva or more likely to be the causative organisms of infection.

3.3.1. Routine Culture of the Eyelid(s)

1. Use a sterile dacron- or polyester-tipped swab that has been moistened in thioglycolate broth.
2. Roll the swab across the anterior lid margins and ulcerated areas of the upper and lower lids of the infected eye.
3. Inoculate onto blood agar and chocolate agar plates by gently rolling on the surface of the agars in an R or L to designate the right and left eyelids, respectively, as shown in Plate 3.

3.3.2. Routine Culture of the Conjunctiva(e):

1. A Kimura spatula is superior for obtaining scrapings for conjunctival cultures and is especially indicated for viral and chlamydial cultures and smears. However, a dacron or polyester swab may be used, moistened in broth as described above.
2. Using a sterile Kimura spatula, scrape across the inferior tarsal conjunctiva and fornix of the infected eye. If a swab is used, swab the area twice as described.
3. Inoculate blood and chocolate agar plates in a zig-zag configuration vertically for the right conjunctiva and in a horizontal manner for the left conjunctiva, as shown in Plate 3. If *Neisseria spp* is suspected, also inoculate a Thayer Martin or New York City agar.
4. In the case of broths and viral or chlamydial transport media, take a fresh scraping after heat sterilization of the Kimura spatula and agitate the tip

immersed in broth, allowing the material to fall into the liquid medium. Place the tip of the applicator into the broth or transport media, swirl several times, then break off swab by stressing it against the internal side of the tube and allow it to fall into the liquid media. Replace the cap and be careful not to tip the thioglycolate tube by placing it in a tube rack, as shown in Figure 3.2.

3.3.3. Cornea Cultures

It is important when culturing corneal ulcers to obtain good specimens for inoculation onto culture medium so that the causative organism can be grown and antibiotic sensitivities obtained. Gram-stained smears from corneal tissue can give immediate information about the causative organism and can guide initial antibiotic treatment; however, it should be kept in mind that cultures are more sensitive in cases of suspect bacterial keratitis. In large ulcers there may be plenty of material available to inoculate both culture media and slides. In smaller ulcers in which the amount of material for sampling is limited, it is advised to inoculate culture media first and then prepare slides for Gram stain, if there is sufficient material available. It is important to prepare slides for special stains if unusual or nonculturable pathogens are suspected.

1. The cornea is anesthetized with a topical anesthetic and a lid speculum is placed.
2. The corneal ulcer is scraped while the patient is sitting at the slit lamp. Using a sterile Kimura spatula, the advancing edge or the necrotic side of the ulcer is debrided in addition to the base of the ulcer.
3. The first scraping obtained from the cornea is then smeared thinly onto two or three clean glass slides. This allows for initial debridement of epithelial surface area, which may have covered the infected area and is best for cellular stains or when unusual pathogens are suspected.
4. The spatula then is resterilized and another debridement is performed. The second scraping is smeared directly onto blood and chocolate agar plates as well as Sabouraud's (if fungus is suspected) or nonnutritive agar (if amoebic keratitis needs to be ruled out).
5. The streaks are made on the agar surface in multiple C shapes as shown in Plate 4.
6. One side of the spatula may be used to inoculate the blood agar plate and the other side for the chocolate agar plate.
7. A sterile dacron-tipped swab moistened in thioglycolate liquid broth medium is then rubbed across the ulcerated area. Care should be exercised so that the lid margin is not touched while swabbing the cornea.
8. The swab tip is then swirled into the thioglycolate liquid and the tip as well as part of the shaft is stressed against the side of tube until broken and allowed to fall into broth. A BHI broth and cooked meat medium may also be inoculated in this same manner and placed upright in a test tube rack as shown in Fig. 3.2.

9. If *Neisseria spp* is suspected, a Thayer Martin or New York City agar should also be inoculated.

3.3.4. Intraocular Fluids (Vitreous Taps, Anterior Chamber Fluid)

1. Obtain cultures from the eyelids and conjunctivae as described previously.
2. Culture the wound or bleb if present.
3. Anesthetize eyelids topically.
4. Anesthetize the eye with a topical or subconjunctival anesthetic in the fornix.
5. Perform a partial-thickness limbal incision.
6. Enter the eye, using a Luer-Lok type or tuberculin syringe (25- to 27-gauge needle).
7. Draw at least 0.5 to 2.0 mL specimen aseptically. Transport the specimen to the laboratory immediately or proceed to inoculate media as in step 8.
8. Inoculate media by placing several drops per plate into the center of the agar surface, as shown in Plate 5. Drop into broth media(s) and two to three glass slides.
9. Fill anterior chamber with sterile balanced salt solution.
10. Obtain a new tuberculin syringe and aspirate vitreous through the limbal opening. Use pars plana approach for phakic patients.
11. Inoculate media and prepare smears as described in step 8.
12. If a vitrectomy is performed the specimen should be processed in the clinical lab by centrifugation of contents then preparing culture and smears from the button or pellet. A filter could also be used by passing fluid through and culturing the filter.

3.3.5. Lacrimal Discharges

1. These types of specimens are considered nonsterile sources and may be obtained by culture transport systems if there is a lot of purulent material present.
2. If discharge is cultured at collection site, the material may be collected with a Kimura spatula, preparing two or three thin smears for staining. If granules or cheesy portions are present, crush these onto the slide.
3. Remove additional discharge using a sterile dacron or polyester swab and streak onto agar surfaces of chocolate and blood agars in an S-shaped figure. An additional blood agar plate should be inoculated for anaerobic culture workup to rule out *Actinomyces spp*.

3.3.6. Abscesses and Deep Wounds

1. If this is an open wound or drainage site, collect and culture in the same manner as for lacrimal discharge because this is a nonsterile source.

2. If this is a closed abscess, aspirate discharge and culture in the same manner as an intraocular fluid because this is a sterile source.

3.3.7. Anaerobic Cultures

This may be done in the operating room or bedside and offers an optimum chance of survival when there is a high degree of suspicion that an anaerobic organism may be the cause of infection. Especially indicated in culture-negative cases to rule out anaerobes.

1. Specimens should be collected and cultured in the same manner as routine bacterial cultures with an additional blood agar plate and thioglycolate medium intended for anaerobic incubation.
2. It is recommended that additional anaerobic cultures of the lids and conjunctiva accompany anaerobic investigation of cornea or intraocular specimens because a large number of anaerobes make up the normal flora of the ocular adnexa.
3. The specimen is collected as indicated by source (i.e., cornea, intraocular fluids, tissue biopsy, conjunctiva, lacrimal), and a blood agar and thioglycolate medium are inoculated for each.
4. Place the blood agar and thioglycolate in a GasPak anaerobic jar (BBL Microbiology Systems, Division of Becton-Dickinson, Cockeysville, MD, U.S.A.) in which a gas-generating envelope, a chemical gas indicator strip, and a catalyst has been placed.
5. The disposable gas-generating envelope is then filled with 10 mL H_2O and the chemical indicator is opened before tightly closing the lid as shown in Figure 3.3.
6. The container is incubated in a 35°C incubator for 72 hours, at which time it may be observed for growth and reincubated for up to 2 weeks, being opened only at 72-hour intervals.

3.3.8. Tissue Biopsies or Keratoplasty Specimens

1. Tissues should be submitted to the microbiology laboratory after excision for routine cultures and so that histopathologic studies may be performed.
2. Inform the microbiologist if unusual pathogens are suspected (i.e., amoebic or microsporidia) so that a portion of tissue can be preserved for possible electron microscopy, and special stains can be used to detect spores or cysts. This is discussed in the following chapter(s).
3. Tissues received in the microbiology laboratory must not be preserved and will be subjected to pulverization by a manual or mechanical tissue grinder. Tissue is placed in a sterile plastic bag with 2 mL broth, and homogenization acts to drive the bacteria from the tissue and into the broth. It is then cultured routinely. It is often best to mince larger tissue specimens into smaller pieces since homogenizing can destroy some organisms.

Figure 3.3
Immediate incubation in an anaer-obic system (BBL GasPak) is im-perative because these sites can be infected with anaerobes with poor air tolerance. Addition of broth anaerobically incubated with plate media facilitates isolation when culture is mixed with aerobes.

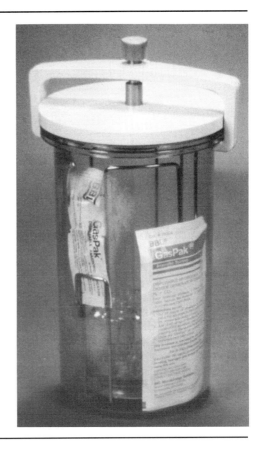

3.3.9. Contact Lenses and Solutions

Cultured in the same manner as tissue and fluids

3.3.10. Donor Corneal Rims and Media

Use of a tissue culture medium containing dextran (McCarey-Kaufman) in the storage of keratoplasty donor material is a routine procedure in eye banks and hospitals. Penicillin and gentamicin or some other antibiotic is often added to minimize contamination and then is stored at 4°C before surgery. Bacteria and fungi may not be inactivated, and therefore many authorities recommend culturing both the corneoscleral tissue (after excision of donor portion) and the liquid holding media. The corneal scleral rim is then set up using routine and fungal culture workups in the microbiology laboratories. This is important because postkeratoplasty infections can have disastrous consequences, as shown in clinical pictures of post-PKP (penetrating keroplasty) fungal keratitis and endophthalmitis (Plates 6 and 7).

3.3.11. Fungal Cultures

1. If a fungal cause is suspected and it is necessary to culture site directly, inoculate a Sabouraud's agar plate in addition to routine bacterial cultures.
2. If *Nocardia spp* or *Actinomyces spp* is suspected, then, in addition to the Sabouraud's agar plate, an additional blood agar and a Lowenstein-Jensen agar slant should be inoculated.
3. Prepare 3 to 4 smears so that a Gram, Giemsa, and special stains such as Calcofluor white or Grocott-Gomori methenamine silver stain for fungus may be performed. These stains will be discussed in section on procedures for staining.

3.3.12. Mycobacterium or Acid-Fast Bacillus Cultures

1. If *M. tuberculosis* or other atypical mycobacteria (as in the immune-compromised host) is suspected, both an egg-based medium (Lowenstein-Jensen slant) and an agar-based medium (Middlebrook 7H10 or 7H11) must be inoculated.
2. Sterile sources such as cornea, intraocular fluids, and most tissue may be directly inoculated.
3. Nonsterile sources such as lacrimal discharge may require decontamination and digestion procedures, which may be performed in the microbiology laboratory.

3.3.13. Parasite Cultures (*Acanthamoeba spp, Naegleria spp,* Microsporidia)

In the last decade we have become increasingly aware of parasites implicated in cases of insidious progressive disciform keratitis mimicking herpes simplex or patchy anterior stromal infiltrates associated with iritis recurrences that fail to respond to bacterial, fungal, or viral therapy. Ring form keratitis with amoebic limbal infiltrates, as seen in cases of *Acanthamoeba spp*, is depicted in Plate 8. This is particularly challenging for the microbiologist and ophthalmologist because there may be several procedures involved in establishing the cause of these infections. There have been at least 700 cases in the literature of acanthamoebic infections and, recently, *Naegleria* too has been implicated in amoebic keratitis. Corneal microsporidiosis is caused by obligate intracellular parasites that may be difficult to diagnose because of their size and frequent inability to stain by conventional methods. Plasmodium (malaria) can be found in the tissue of the eye using hematoxylin and eosin stain, as seen in Plate 9, and birefringence of hemozoin (malarial pigment) can be viewed under polarized light, as shown in Plate 10. Other parasitemias include cysticerci of *Taenia solium, Loa Loa* (African eye worm), *Toxocara spp* (often mistaken for cancer of the eye), and toxoplasmosis.

Parasitic involvement should be included in the differential diagnosis of the immune-compromised host (particularly in cases of acquired immune deficiency syndrome [AIDS]), contact lens wearers, severely scarred or vascularized cornea or conjunctivae, and in cases of trauma or exposure to farm animals or insects.

The following is a guideline to specimen requirements for procedures used in establishing the diagnosis of parasitemia, particularly amoebic or microsporidial keratitis. More detailed information is contained in the sections for culture, stained smears, and transmission electron microscopy. Because these are unusual isolates, some media or fixatives are not described here and may vary.

1. The preferred method of specimen collection is tissue biopsy or keratoplasty. However, cysts of *Acanthamoeba spp* and *Naegleria spp* as well as spores from various Microsporidia can sometimes be found in a corneal or conjunctival scraping. One should keep in mind that the tendency of these organisms to be found deep in the stromal layers of the tissue may yield negative results if one only scrapes the surface epithelial cells. Microsporidia spores and plasmodia are more likely to be found in corneal or conjunctival scrapings than are *Acanthamoeba spp* or *Naegleria spp*.
2. Divide tissue into four portions if possible. If performing a scraping, transfer to four clean glass slides for staining by Gram, Giemsa, Grocott-Gomori methenamine silver, and calcofluor white (or other special stains such as trichrome, periodic acid-Schiff, or hematoxylin and eosin).
3. One portion or scraping should be placed on a nonnutrient agar plate and another portion sent to microbiology for routine culture and special stains.
4. One portion of tissue (contact lenses may be done in the same manner) should be fixed in formalin and embedded in paraffin for histopathologic studies.
5. One portion preserved by 2% glutaraldehyde fixation used in many institutions or aldehyde-osmium rapid fixative (described in transmission electron microscopy section).
6. Another portion may be needed for *in vitro* tissue culture studies and preserved in a fixative such as Hank's balanced salt solution if your laboratory or reference laboratory has the facilities to perform tissue culture of Microsporidia and you wish to identify to the genera or species level by demonstration in culture. Prepare as follows:

Hank's Balanced Salt Solution:
For each liter of solution, prepare solutions 1 and 2 separately and label them "solution 1" and "solution 2," respectively. Dissolve the ingredients for each in approximately 500 mL reagent-grade water.
Solution 1:
NaCl .... 80.0 g
KCl .... 4.0 g
$CaCl_2$ .... 1.4 g
$MgSO_4$ .... 2.0 g
Solution 2:
$Na_2HPO_4 \cdot 12H_2O$ .... 1.52 g
KH_2PO_4 .... 0.6 g
Glucose .... 10.0 g
Phenol Red 1% .... 16.0 mL
Slowly add solution 1 to solution 2 while stirring. Adjust the final volume to 1000 mL (1 L) with reagent-grade water. This is a 10× solution that should be sterilized, preferably by filter sterilization. If steam steriliza-

tion is desired, dilute to a 1× solution first with reagent-grade water and prepare aliquots in test tubes. Steam sterilize for 10 minutes at 10 lb/in^2 (110°C). Do not sterilize for a longer period or at a higher temperature because this may carmelize the glucose. Just before use, the 1× solution must be buffered by the addition of 12.5 mL 2.8% NaHCO$_3$ solution per liter.

7. Note on the request form that amoebiosis or microsporidiosis is suspected and communicate with the clinical laboratory before taking cultures and smears to be sure that they are able to perform the necessary tests or to work out the logistics of transferring material to an outside reference or research laboratory.

3.3.14. Impression Cytology Collection and Protocol for Fixation

1. General principle
Calibrated precut cellulose acetate filter papers (Millipore) are placed on selected areas of the conjunctiva in a configuration that will permit accurate identification of anatomic location when performing the stain procedure. Figure 3.4. shows a schematic illustration of filter application. The filter papers are then peeled off, thereby taking with them an impression of the surface epithelial layer impregnated within the pores of the filter paper. These are stored in a cytologic preservative before being stained by Gill's Modified Papanicolaou method.

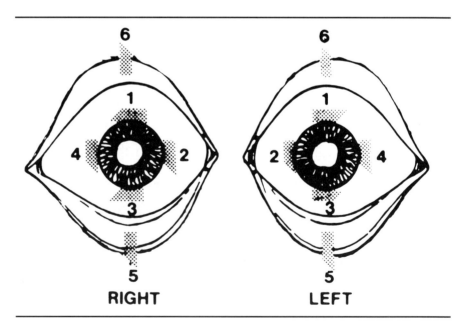

Figure 3.4
Illustration of filter paper orientation when applied to the conjunctiva used in impression cytology procedures.

Once stained, the number of goblet cells as well as changes in epithelial cells can be assessed.

2. Additional materials required
Hawp 304 cellulose acetate filter paper (Millipore)
24- or 48-well plastic tissue culture plates
Lid speculum
Tying forceps
Topical anesthetic
Sterile dacron or polyester swabs
Facial tissues
Paper stick-on labels
Plastic squirt bottle for fixative storage
Portable alcohol burner or bacterial incinerator
Diagram of impression filter paper orientation (Figure 3.4)

3. Fixative
Prepared by combining the following reagents:

1. Glacial acetic acid .... 10 mL
2. 37% formaldehyde.. 10 mL
3. 70% ethanol .... 200 mL

Mix by swirling and store in a plastic squeeze/squirt bottle.

4. Procedure
This will take approximately 15 minutes.

1. Write patient's name, identification number, date, and time on a label and affix it to the cover of a tissue culture plate. A computer-generated label also may be used.
2. Place 1 to 2 drops topical anesthetic in the right eye.
3. Insert a lid speculum into the right eye.
4. Use the tying forceps to place a filter paper in position 1 on the superior limbus, as indicated in diagram Figure 3.4. The pointed end of the filter paper is used to grasp with tying forceps.
5. Apply slight pressure using the forceps, gently but firmly, in all four quadrants and in the center of the paper to ensure full contact with the paper. This should last 3 to 5 seconds. Be sure that excessive tearing does not prevent the paper from making contact with the surface of epithelial. If paper becomes saturated with tears, discard and repeat. If necessary, use a swab or tissue to dry up the lacrimal lake, but do not allow this to touch the area where the filter paper is intended to make contact.
6. Grasping the pointed end, peel off slowly, as shown in Figure 3.5.
7. Place into the first well of the tissue culture plate, as shown in Figure 3.6.
8. Repeat steps 4 through 8 for positions 2, 3, and 4 of the diagram, always placing the filter paper into separate wells corresponding to the position number.

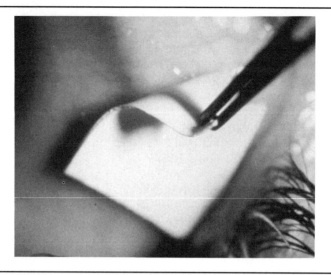

Figure 3.5
The filter papers are peeled off, taking with them an impression of the epithelial sur-
face now trapped within the pores of the paper. Courtesy of Barbara Blodi, M.D.,
W. K. Kellogg Eye Center, University of Michigan, Ann Arbor, Michigan.

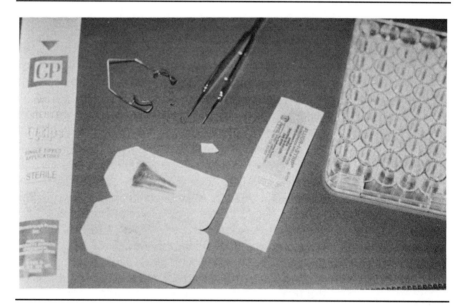

Figure 3.6
Materials used in specimen collection and ophthalmic examination. The filter papers
are placed immediately into wells of a tissue culture plate before being filled with fixa-
tive. Courtesy of Barbara Blodi, M.D., W. K. Kellogg Eye Center, University of
Michigan, Ann Arbor, Michigan.

9. Remove the lid speculum to perform procedure on the lids.
10. Pull the inferior lid down and place filter paper in position 5, and repeat steps 5 through 7.
11. Evert the upper lid and place filter paper in position 6 (this may require assistance) and repeat steps 5 through 7.
12. Place 2 to 3 drops of anesthetic into the left eye.
13. Follow positions indicated for the left eye and repeat steps 3 through 11.
14. Fill all wells with fixative and replace culture plate cover. Fixation is complete in 10 minutes, but filter papers may be stored for several days this way until ready to perform staining. Be sure that wells do not dry up and replenish periodically with additional fixative if needed.

3.3.15. Conjunctival Scraping Procedure for *Chlamydia* or Cytology Smears

This procedure may be used when only smears are required or when culturing and performing Micro-Trak Direct Fluorescent Antibody (Syva C., San Jose, CA) tests for *Chlamydia*. Smears prepared from these sites are optimal for conjunctival cell morphology when *Chlamydia* is suspected and when isolation of this organism is desired. This procedure can also be used for cytology requests such as vernal conjunctivitis and others.

Upper conjunctiva
1. Use a sterile Kimura spatula or one that may be flamed or bacti-incinerated to red hot and allowed to cool immediately before use.
2. Label slides with name and patient identification number, using a lead pencil.
3. Instill 2 to 3 drops of a topical (nonbactericidal) anesthetic into the eye.
4. Have the patient look downward and evert the upper lid to expose the tarsal plate of the conjunctiva.
5. Gently scrape the epithelial surface, keeping at least 2 to 3 mm away from the lid margin.
6. Spread the sample onto the center of a precleaned glass slide to obtain a thin smear. Turn the spatula over to spread the remaining sample either on the same slide or a second slide or Micro-Trak sample slide into two individual circles.
7. Allow to air dry and fix immediately in appropriate fixative (methanol for Gram stain and others, acetone for Micro-Trak, Papanicolaou fixative for cytology, etc.) or transport to the laboratory if able to do so within 15 to 20 minutes. Indicate whether smear is fixed or unfixed.

Lower tarsal conjunctiva
Have the patient look upward and pull down the lower lid. Repeat steps 1, 2, and 5 through 7.

BIBLIOGRAPHY

Al-Hazzaa SAF, Tabbara KF: Bacterial keratitis following penetrating keratoplasty. Ophthalmology 1988;95(11):1504–1508.

Al-Mutlaq F, Byrne-Rhodes KA, Tabbara KF: *Neisseria meningitidis* conjunctivitis in children. Am J Ophthalmol 1987;104:280–282.

Blodi BA, Byrne KA, Tabbara KF: Goblet cell population among patients with inactive trachoma. Int Ophthalmol J 1988;12(1):41–45.

Davis RM, Font RL, Keisler MS, Shadduck JA. Corneal microsporidiosis. Ophthalmology 1990;97(7):953–957.

Friedberg DN, Stenson SM, Orenstein JM, et al.: Microsporidial keratoconjunctivitis in acquired immunodeficiency syndrome. Arch Ophthalmol 1990;108:504–508.

Fritsche TR, Gautom RK, Seyedirashti S, et al.: Occurrence of bacterial endosymbionts in *Acanthamoeba spp* isolated from corneal and environmental specimens and contact lenses. J Clin Microbiol 1993;31(5):1122–1126.

Gangadharam PRJ, Lanier JD, Jones DB: Keratitis due to *Mycobacterium chelonei*. Tubercle 1978;59:55–60.

Garcia LS: Freshwater amoebae. Clinical Microbiology Newsletter. New York: Elsevier, 1983;5(16):107–114.

Hidayat AA, Nalbandian RM, Sammons DW, et al.: The diagnostic histopathologic features of ocular malaria. Ophthalmology 1993;100(8)1183–1186.

Jones DB, Liesegang TJ, Robinson NM: Laboratory diagnosis of ocular infections. In Washington JA (ed): Cumitech 13: Cumulative techniques and procedures in clinical microbiology. Washington, DC: American Society for Microbiology, May 1981.

Liesegang TJ: Atypical ocular toxocariasis. J Pediatr Ophthalmol 1977;14:349–353.

McNatt J, Allen SD, Wilson LA, Dowell VR: Anaerobic flora of the normal human conjunctival sac. Arch Ophthalmol 1978;96:1448–1450.

Nash P, Krenz MM: Culture media, Hank's balanced salt solution. Chapter 121. In Balows A, Hausler WJ, Herrmann KL, et al. (eds.): Manual of clinical microbiology, 5th Edition, 1991:1249. American Society for Microbiology, Washington, D.C.

Smith RE, Nobe JR: Eye infections. In Finegold SM, George WL (eds): Anaerobic infections in humans. New York: Academic Press, 1989.

Smolin G, Tabbara KF, Witcher J: Infectious diseases of the eye. Baltimore: Williams & Wilkins, 1984.

Tabbara KF: Ocular toxoplasmosis. Int Ophthalmol J 1990;14:349–351.

Tabbara KF: Toxoplasmosis and toxocariasis. In Practical management of macular diseases: A text and atlas. Boston: W.B. Saunders. In press.

Tseng SCG: Impression cytology and squamous metaplasia. Ophthalmology 1985;92:728–733.

Yee RW, Tio FO, Martinez JA, et al.: Resolution of microsporidial epithelial keratopathy in a patient with AIDS. Ophthalmology 1991:98(2):196–201.

Staining Procedures for Microscopy

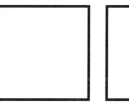

4

There are a myriad of stains (and modifications of those) currently available in the clinical laboratory and an unlimited number of manufacturers willing to supply them, further testament to the important role microscopic techniques play in presumptive and definitive diagnosis of infectious disease. In many cases, stained smears give important clues and provide the basis of presumptive diagnosis on the day of specimen receipt. Choices of initial stains in unusual ocular infections can be critical in establishing the diagnosis. In culture they may be essential for identifying the offending pathogen. The cytology may aid in determining whether bacterial pathogens are normal flora that may be colonizing the site or causing the infection. In the case of unculturable or nonviable organisms, they may be the only resource available for determining the cause of those infections. Knowledge of the factors involved in stains and the organism's ability to take up or reject those stains is the basis of their use in the clinical or research laboratory. Other types of microscopy may not rely on stain but on techniques in light, fluorescence, and transmission electron microscopy. With the use of monoclonal antibody procedures using known organisms, we can expand the scope of initial smears to include not only the organism present in the smear but also the probability that it is there. The complexity and fixation requirements of these preparations requires the ophthalmologist and microbiologist to become familiar with certain ocular disease processes so that they can make the best choice before specimen collection and be aware of how to proceed once certain factors are unveiled during workup in the laboratory. Although some of these stains or microscopy procedures may be ages old (despite some modifications), their application for bacteria, fungi, parasites, and certain cytology may be new to the reader. Therefore, we have included common and uncommon stains and techniques, including their modifications as they apply to pathogens and cytology of ocular disease. To see the results of certain stains, one can refer to the legend and color atlas after this section. When possible, these color plates are referred to in the individual staining or microscopy procedure. The stains are, generally, grouped by the type of microscopy and include their application in the investigation of a particular disease. When appropriate, we discuss alternative stains that may be necessary to establish the diagnosis of unusual pathogens. In many cases definitive diagnosis of a disease process can be achieved by combining certain techniques and demonstration of these before or after detection in culture. Initial smears and direct preparation of isolated organisms may require similar fixation and preparation for further testing by methods in microscopy. However, the microbiologist should be aware that some of the biochemicals contained in selective medias may affect the staining reactions of certain organisms. Therefore, whenever possible, organisms for staining should be taken from culture material without the addition of biochemicals, including antibiotics. This may require subculture to a nonchemical media not containing antibiotics before staining or when atypical reactions are observed. Many broths, including thioglycolate, affect the Gram stain results of smears taken from these media. This is particularly true of gram-positive rods, which very often appear gram negative. Because smears need to be taken from both initially if this is the only positive culture, it is necessary to repeat these once plate growth is achieved. *Bacillus spp* is one of the great pretenders because of its appearance as gram negative in broth and growth on selective media. When carried through culture workup it is nonsaccharolytic, often being mistaken for *Pseudomonas spp* without being discovered for several days if the Gram stain is not repeated. So, just to be aware of odd characteristics can save the patient and hospital unnecessary expense and inappropriate antibiotic treatment, which in the long run far outweighs the time or cost of repeating stain procedures. In this day of cost-productive efficiencies, certain tests may be eliminated, but, when reducing steps in the workup of ocular smears and cultures, one needs to be aware of the large number of possible isolates and the seriousness of these infections.

4.1. LIGHT MICROSCOPY: STAINS AND UNSTAINED TECHNIQUES

The following procedures may be performed using a standard light microscope with 10×, 40× to 50×, and 100× objectives. The use of a 10× ocular is equivalent to a magnification of 100 times, 400 to 500 times, and 1000 times magnification, respectively, of a particular object under examination. This is adequate to identify most bacteria, parasites, fungi, and cells. Additional equipment that may be necessary for light microscopy includes a polarizing system and a phase contrast option or darkfield for the examination of syphilis and other organisms. Many fluorescence techniques, discussed later, negate the need for darkfield but some laboratories still prefer to use this when a fluorescence microscope is not available. Variations in techniques are explained when pertinent. Good quality control demands that a microscope be calibrated regularly and light condenser be used to provide bright field for microscopy.

4.1.1. Conventional Gram Stain

Purpose

The Gram-stained smear is the primary and most important bacteriologic technique. It provides essential information as to the quality of the specimen and it categorizes most bacteria into one of two groups, "gram positive" and "gram negative," based on staining characteristics defined by the structures of their cell walls. It is primarily used to stain direct smears, tissue, and exudates when information concerning the presence or absence of microorganisms is desired. Important clues such as intracellular organisms, as seen in Figure 4.1 of gram-negative diplococci in *Neisseria meningitidis* conjunctivitis, and quantity of certain organisms, as presented in Plate 11 of *Haemophilus influenzae* conjunctivitis, can determine whether bacterial pathogens from ocular sites with normal flora are colonizing the site or causing an infection. Some cells can be determined by Gram stain alone, such as polymorphonuclear leukocytes (neu-

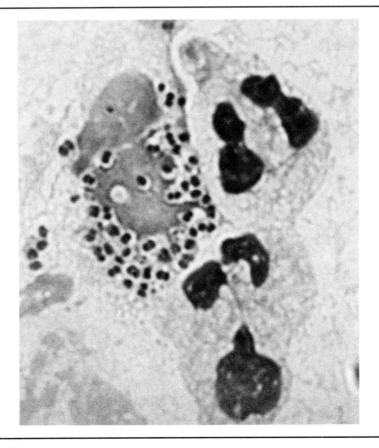

Figure 4.1
Gram-negative intracellular diplococci characteristic of the Neisseria spp *in conjunctivitis of a child. Gram stain, 1,000× magnification.*

trophils), and their number in comparison with the epithelial and mononuclear types of white cells can provide additional clues to the cause of infection, that is, bacterial or viral. Occasional strains of clostridia, staphylococci, and streptococci can secrete toxins that may destroy neutrophils, so one should note this when observing a dominance of one of these organisms and a distinct neutropenia. This can yield a rapid presumptive diagnosis and guide antibiotic therapy while culture results are pending. During antibiotic therapy, organisms may be detected while culture results are negative or an organism dominating culture plate is minor in smears. Because it takes a large number of organisms to be seen on smears, trust the Gram stain because certain organisms grow better *in vitro* or could be contaminants. Presence on Gram stain and no growth on standard culture media also may signal the presence of anaerobic organisms. Virtually all identification procedures and decisions for culture workups begin with Gram stain and again when growth is achieved in culture.

General principle

Gram stain effectively divides bacterial species into two large groups: those that take up the basic dye, crystal violet (gram positive) and those that allow the crystal violet dye to wash off with the decolorizer alcohol or acetone (gram negative). It involves preparing the material with a methanol fixative (methanol fixation is superior to heat because it preserves cellular background and causes less distortion of cells and bacteria and a better Gram reaction overall). After fixation, crystal violet stain is applied, staining all bacteria a blue-purple color. Gram's iodine is applied to chemically bond the alkaline dye to the cell wall. The decolorization step distinguishes the two, probably because gram-negative bacterial cells are abundant in lipids, the alcohol-acetone increases the permeability of the cell wall, and the alkaline dye washes away (gram negative). The increased amount of teichoic acid residues found in other bacterial cell walls work to enhance binding of crystal violet (gram positive). In the second step, in which the counterstain is applied, the bacteria and other cells that were made colorless take up the safranin or basic fuchsin dye, turning red or pink in contrast to the darkly stained gram positives as seen in Figure 4.2. of staphylococcal (gram-positive) keratitis and Plate 12, showing gram-negative rods in *Moraxella* keratitis.

Procedure

1. It is recommended to purchase these reagents from a supply vendor rather than to prepare from powdered reagents, to maintain consistency and quality control. If this is not possible, however, the following procedure can be used:

   Prepare reagents as follows:
   A. Crystal Violet Solution:
      Crystal violet (90% dye content)..10 g
      dissolved in absolute methyl alcohol................................. 500 mL
   B. Iodine Solution:
      Iodine crystals... 6 g
      Potassium iodine... 12 g

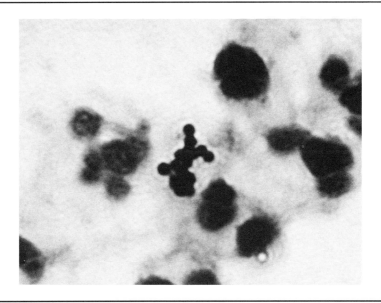

Figure 4.2
*Gram-positive cocci in cluster found in staphylococcal keratitis. Gram stain, 1,000×
magnification.*

	Distilled water	1800 mL

C. Decolorizer:

	Acetone	400 mL
	95% Ethanol	1200 mL

D. Counterstain:

	Safranin (99% dye content)	10 g
	Distilled water	1000 mL

2. Fix smears by flooding with methanol, allowing this to stay on air-dried smears for 2 minutes.
3. Place air-dried smear on staining rack and flood slide with solution of crystal violet 30 to 60 seconds.
4. Rinse slide with deionized water, taking care not to spray directly on smear, but flood gently so as not to wash material off.
5. Flood slide with solution of iodine and allow to remain for at least 60 seconds.
6. Rinse slide with water and shake off excess.
7. Flood slide with decolorizer for 10 seconds and rinse immediately.
8. Flood slide with safranin or basic fuchsin counterstain and leave on for 20 to 30 seconds.
9. Rinse slide with deionized water and allow to air dry or place on heat block (45°C).
10. Examine microscopically under 10× or 40× to 50× objectives to search for good areas (where cells can be found) and possible larger fungal ele-

ments then under oil immersion 100× (1000× magnification) brightfield for bacteria, white cells, or other structures. Read the entire smear and record the findings.

Quality control and interpretation

It is a good idea to prepare control slides from saline suspensions of gram-negative rods and gram-positive cocci to run each time a test slide is performed. The bacteria that retain the blue-purple color of the primary stain are reported as gram positive, and those that lose the primary stain and only pick up the red or pink counterstain are reported as gram negative. Further morphologic characteristics are also noted such as shape (bacilli, cocci, diplococci, etc.) and if spores are observed, etc. The key to a good Gram stain is having a thin smear. Thick smears may cause distortion and variable Gram staining caused by lack of penetration of decolorizer or interfere with stain absorption because of crowding of organisms.

Quantitation of bacteria and cells

Quantitation of bacteria and cells from stained smears should include a rapid estimation of bacterial morphotype and cellular type (i.e., polymorphonuclear, mononuclear, and epithelial cells) and a description of the quality of these as in disintegrating cells and moderate to heavy cellular debris. Scan the entire smear in random areas before deciding on the quantity of each element. Generally,

very few or occasional = one or two in some but not every field
few to light = one to five elements in most fields
several or moderate = five to ten per field
many or heavy = more than ten per field

If bacteria or polymorphs are absent or the physician has indicated a suspect organism that is not present on smear, you should also note this at the time of reporting.

Limitations

Some bacteria or other elements may be affected by antibiotics, or if from broth or selective media cultures, and may not exhibit normal staining properties. These can include gram-positive rods such as *Bacillus spp* and *Clostridium spp*, which may demonstrate spores or lose their ability to hold crystal violet stain and may appear gram negative or variable. Certain other bacteria such as *Streptococcus pneumoniae* may contain a capsule that washes off and can appear as gram-negative cocci. The shape of a capsule can sometimes be seen against the cellular background, as shown in Plate 13. Anaerobic gram-negative rods often stain palely and may have a club shape, as with *Bacteroides spp* seen in Plate 14. Fungal elements do not always stain by Gram stain, but may also be seen against the background or stain partially, as in Plate 15. Suspect smears should be restained by Grocott-Gomori methenamine silver or with a Calcofluor white fluorescence method when in doubt. This is also true for suspect parasites that may be seen on initial smears.

BIBLIOGRAPHY

Al-Hemidan A, Byrne-Rhodes KA, Tabbara KF: *Bacillus cereus* panophthalmitis associated with intraocular gas bubble. Br J Ophthalmol 1989; 73:25–28.

Al-Mutlaq F, Byrne-Rhodes KA, Tabbara KF: *Neisseria meningitidis* conjunctivitis in children. Am J Ophthalmol 1987; 104:280–282.

Baron EJ, Peterson L, Finegold SM (eds.): Bailey and Scott's diagnostic microbiology, 9th Edition. St. Louis: C. V. Mosby, 1994.

Mangels JI, Cox ME, Lindberg LH: Methanol fixation: An alternative to heat fixation of smears before staining. Diagn Microbiol Infect Dis 1984; 2:129–137.

Wegner D: Gram stains, Session 47, 1993 Northwest Symposium by the Pacific Area Resource Office of the National Laboratory Training Network and Centers for Disease Control.

4.1.2 Giemsa Stained Preparations

Purpose

Giemsa stain is used for the permanent preparation of smears for detection of chlamydial inclusion bodies and cellular changes relating to trachoma. In addition, the presence or predominance of certain types of inflammatory cells as well as changes in epithelial cells may indicate other disease states. Direct microscopy of epithelial cell scrapings may be useful in diagnosing chlamydial infections and, because of the staining properties of eosinophils and other cells, it may be beneficial in the diagnoses of bacterial, allergic, parasitic, or viral cell immune responses. Giemsa stain is the cytologic stain most commonly used for ophthalmic specimens because, in addition to demonstrating the cell types present, it best demonstrates intracytoplasmic inclusion bodies. Intranuclear inclusions are not seen in smears stained with Giemsa because the nuclear chromatin stains heavily and obscures the inclusion. Hematoxylin and eosin (H & E) or preferably Papanicolaou stain can be used to stain intranuclear inclusions.

Principle

Giemsa stain combines chemically with bacterial protoplasm. Chlamydiae are rich in nucleic acid, bearing negative charges as phosphate groups that combine readily with positively charged basic or analine dyes. Acidic dyes do not stain bacterial cells and hence can be used to stain the background a contrasting color.

Reagents

Many manufacturer-prepared medias are available, and package inserts should be consulted. If these are not available, or if preferred, the following procedure may be used to prepare reagents:

Preparation of buffered water for Giemsa stain:
Solution A: 0.067 mol/L disodium phosphate (Na_2HPO_4)
Na$_2$HPO$_4$... 9.5 g
Distilled water... 1 liter
Place the phosphate salt in a 1000-mL volumetric flask; add a small amount of distilled water to dissolve, then dilute to the mark with distilled water.

Solution B: monosodium phosphate (NaH_2PO_4 $2H_2O$)

Monosodium phosphate .... 9.2 g

Distilled water.. 1.0 liter

Place the phosphate salt in a 1000-mL volumetric flask; add a small amount of distilled water to dissolve, then dilute to the mark with distilled water.

NOTE: These solutions keep indefinitely in a refrigerator in capped or stoppered glass bottles.

Working Solution: pH 7.0

Solution A .... 61.1 mL

Solution B .... 38.9 mL

Distilled water.. 900.0 mL

Staining procedure — rapid method

1. Fix slide in 95% methanol for 5 minutes.
2. Place 6 to 7 drops of Giemsa stock stain on slide.
3. Add 18 to 20 drops buffered water (pH 7.0). A green sheen should appear on the slide.
4. Allow stain to remain on slide in the incubator at 37°C for 15 minutes or in the microwave oven for 5 to 7 minutes at 50% power; however, this should be experimented with.
5. Rinse off the stain using distilled water.
6. Allow slide to air dry.
7. Examine slide under a brightfield light microscope.

Staining procedure: 1-hour method (preferred method)

1. Fix slide in 95% methanol for 5 minutes.
2. Prepare fresh stain solution in a Coplin staining jar.
   a. Place 2 mL stock Giemsa stain in the bottom of the Coplin jar.
   b. Add buffered water to within one-half inch from the top (approximately 70 mL).
3. Incubate slide in stain at 35°C to 37°C for 60 minutes.
4. Differentiate using two changes of 95% ethanol.
5. Rinse in tap water.
6. Allow slide to air dry.
7. Examine slide under a brightfield light microscope.

Interpretation

Red Blood Cells: are pinkish to pink-blue color.

Mononuclear Cells: nucleus is round, deep purple, and cytoplasm is sky blue to darker blue.

Eosinophils: nucleus stains deep purple to purple-blue, granules appear bright and are orange to pink-orange in color.

Polymorphonuclear Leukocytes: nucleus is deep purple to purple-blue, granules are a pink to pink-blue color.

Quantitation of certain cell types should be performed as in a white blood count differential and measured per 100 epithelial cells using a standard hematologic cell differential counter as demonstrated in Figure 4.3. Inflammatory cells and red blood cells with epithelial cells are shown in Plate 16. The intensity of the cellular response and its significance is determined by the predominant type of inflammatory cell as described in the following chapter, entitled Cytology. Other morphology is also reported such as separate or sheets of epithelial and mucus strands or melanin granules if present. Inclusion bodies may be seen within the cytoplasm of epithelial cells, and elementary bodies also may be present outside the cells, as seen in Plate 17. These stain blue to purple with Giemsa stain.

Other morphology associated with *Chlamydia trachomatis* infection is detailed in Chapter 5: Cytology.

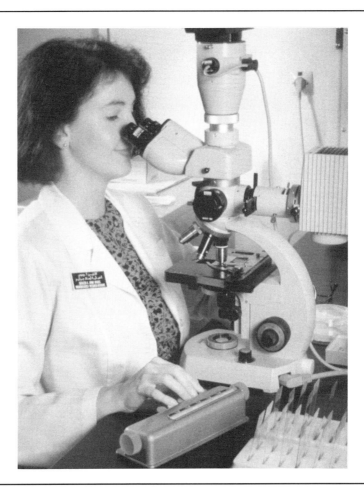

Figure 4.3
K. Byrne demonstrates microscopy using a cell counter, camera attachment, and other options available for use with standard Kohler illuminated microscopes.

Quality control
1. Peripheral blood smears should exhibit appropriate staining characteristics of cell types as just described.
2. If the smear does not exhibit these staining characteristics, fresh stain is prepared and the procedure is repeated with new control smear and patient's smear(s).
3. If bacteria appear in control smear, the buffer may have become contaminated and should not be used.

BIBLIOGRAPHY

Balows A, Hausler WJ, Herrmann KL, et al.: Giemsa stains. In Manual of clinical microbiology, 5th Edition. Washington D.C.: American Society For Microbiology. 1991:1304–1305.

Jones DB, Liesegang TJ, Robinson NM: Laboratory diagnosis of ocular infections. In CUMITECH 13: Cumulative techniques and procedures in clinical microbiology. Washington DC: American Society of Microbiology, May 1981: 12–18.

Washington JA (ed.): Laboratory procedures in clinical microbiology. New York: Springer-Verlag, 1981:83–84.

4.1.3. The Diff-Quik Stain

Purpose
The Diff-Quik stain comes closest to meeting the requirements of a simple, fast, differential stain. This stain may be used for the detection of bacteria, fungi, and chlamydial inclusions, as well as for the identification of various cell types and exudates that may be found in an eye scraping. The reagents are stable at room temperature, so the solutions kept in Coplin jars need not be changed for a month or longer, depending on workload.

Principle
The Diff-Quik stain is manufactured by HARLECO, a division of American Hospital Supply Corporation U.S.A. This polychromatic stain is a modification of the original time-consuming Romanowsky-type stains using the aniline methylene blue and eosin dyes.

Procedure
Diff-Quick comes in a package of three bottled solutions, and the stain may be performed on prepared smears by dipping the slides in stain aliquots poured off into 3 coplin jars as follows:

1. Fixative: .... 5 dips
2. Solution I (an eosin dye) .... 5 dips
3. Solution II (a basic dye) .... 5 dips

Finally, rinse slides gently in deionized water and allow to air dry. Examine slides under brightfield light microscopy at 1000× and oil immersion.

Interpretation
Bacteria stain blue, and fungi may stain variably or partially but are visible against the cellular background. The staining characteristics of inflammatory cells closely resemble that for Giemsa stain.

Quality control
It is recommended that a peripheral blood smear be used as a control to assure the quality of the technique and stability of stains.

Limitations
1. The colors are not fully saturated and therefore are not as intense as a longer staining method.
2. There is a tendency for some areas to stain less than others.
3. Identification of chlamydial inclusions may require restaining by the longer Giemsa method, because they may not be basophilic as desired.

BIBLIOGRAPHY

Byrne-Rhodes KA: The Diff-Quik Stain. Saudi Bull Ophthalmol 1987; 2(1):24.
Rogers, Plotkin SA: A rapid stain for ocular cytology. J Pediatr Ophthalmol 1974; 11:158–160.

4.1.4. Kinyoun Procedure for Staining Acid-Fast Bacilli

Purpose
Certain organisms, particularly *Mycobacterium spp*, do not stain by conventional methods. These are aerobic, non–spore-forming, nonmotile bacteria that are acid fast. Acid-fast examinations for the diagnosis of mycobacterial infections and actinomycetes are simple, rapid, and have a high specificity, although they are not as sensitive as the Auramine-Rhodamine fluorescence method.

Principle
In Kinyoun's method, the concentration of basic fuchsin and phenol is increased, avoiding the need for heat. It works by fixing the carbol fuchsin within the lipid cell walls of mycobacteria (Balows et al. 1991).

Procedure
Prepare stock reagents as follows:

1. Kinyoun carbol-fuchsin stain (Baron et al. 1994):
   Basic fuchsin (dry) .... 4 g
   Phenol (crystallized) .... 8 g
   95% Ethanol .... 0.20 mL
   Deionized water .... 100 mL
2. Acid-Alcohol:
   95% Ethanol .... 97 mL

       Hydrochloric acid (concentrated) .... 3 mL
3. Methylene blue counterstain:
       Methylene blue.. 0.3 g
       Deionized water .... 100 mL

   a. Heat-fix smears by flaming or with an 85°C slide warming plate and run along with test smears, one prepared with positive acid-fast bacilli and another smear that does not exhibit acid-fast staining.
   b. Place slides on a staining rack and flood with Carbol-fuchsin solution for 2 to 5 minutes. Do not heat.
   c. Wash gently in running water.
   d. Decolorize with acid-alcohol decolorizer, allowing it to run off the slide until dye no longer washes off slide.
   e. Wash gently in running water.
   f. Counterstain for 30 seconds with Brilliant Green or Methylene Blue.
   g. Wash gently with tap water and air dry.

Interpretation

Acid-fast organisms stain red, and other organisms, as well as cellular elements, stain blue or the contrasting color of the counterstain used, as shown in Plate 18. Other atypical or nontuberculous bacteria also resemble *Mycobacterium tuberculosis* and may be pathogenic in immune-compromised individuals (Saubolle 1989).

Quality control

Control slides should exhibit expected acid-fast, positive staining, and negative control slide should not contain acid-fast organisms. If this is not the case, repeat procedure with fresh patient and control slides.

BIBLIOGRAPHY

Balows A, Hausler WJ, Herrmann KL, et al.: Manual of clinical microbiology, 5th Edition. Washington, D.C.: American Society for Microbiology, 1991: 313, 1308.
Baron EJ, Peterson L, Finegold SM (eds.): Bailey and Scott's diagnostic microbiology, 9th Edition. St. Louis: C. V. Mosby, 1994, Chapter 42:607.
Saubolle MA: Nontuberculous mycobacteria as agents of human disease in the United States. Clin Microbiol News 1989; 11(15):113–117.

4.1.5. Ziehl-Neelsen Acid-Fast Stain for Tissue

Purpose

For the staining of mycobacteria, Actinomycetes, and coccidian parasites such as *Cryptosporidium spp*, which may be characterized by their acid-fast staining properties.

Principle

The cell walls of some parasites and bacteria contain long-chain mycolic acids (fatty acids), which have the property of resistance to destaining of basic dyes by acid alcohol, hence the term *acid-fast*. The Ziehl-Neelsen requires heat to enter the wax-containing cell wall, allowing the organism to be stained.

Procedure

All ingredients are available from many chemical suppliers. Prepare as follows:

1. Carbol Fuchsin solution (Baron et al. 1994; Balows et al. 1991):
   Basic Fuchsin.. 0.5 g
   Phenol crystals (melted).. 2.5 mL
   Ethanol 95%... 5 mL
   Deionized water .... 50 mL
   Dissolve fuchsin in alcohol, then add phenol and water. Let stand for 24 to 72 hours. Filter through fine paper to remove any acid-fast bacilli before use. Store at room temperature.
2. Acid Alcohol Decolorizer:
   95% Ethanol.. 97 mL
   Concentrated hydrochloric acid .... 3 mL
   Add hydrochloric acid to ethanol slowly.
3. Methylene blue (working solution):
   Methylene blue chloride... 0.5 g
   Glacial acetic acid .... 0.5 mL
   Distilled or deionized water.. 100 mL
Mix in a clean bottle. Filter twice before use.

Fix prepared tissue slides on a heated surface of at least 60°C for 10 minutes. Flood smears with carbol fuchsin and heat to almost boiling by performing the procedure on a heated platform. Let sit for 5 minutes without drying. Wash in deionized or distilled water (distilled is preferred because tap water may contain other acid-fast bacilli). Flood with decolorizer for 1 minute. Continue to flood if slide still runs red. Rinse thoroughly with water to remove excess dye. Flood slides with methylene blue counterstain and leave on 1 minute. Rinse slides; do not blot dry. Dehydrate with 95% alcohol and absolute alcohol. Mount in Permount. Examine by brightfield light microscopy; first with $400\times$ to $500\times$ magnification and confirm at $1000\times$ with oil immersion.

Interpretation

Acid-fast organisms (including Actinomycetes) appear bright red, whereas erythrocytes appear yellow-orange and background tissue stains pale blue, as shown in Plate 19.

Quality control

A positive Actinomycetes or *Cryptosporidium* prepared slide should be run along with the patient slide for comparison. A negative slide should also be run to detect contaminants. If expected results are not achieved, both test and control should be repeated.

REFERENCES

Balows A, Hausler WJ, Herrmann KL, et al.: Manual of clinical microbiology, 5th Edition. Washington, D.C.: American Society for Microbiology, 1991: 1313.

Baron EJ, Peterson L, Finegold SM (eds.): Bailey and Scott's diagnostic microbiology, 9th Edition. St. Louis: C. V. Mosby, 1994, p. 607, Chapter 42.

4.1.6. Trichrome Stain for Parasites, Amoebic Keratitis, and Spores of Microsporidia

Purpose
For the detection of parasitic cysts, spores, and protozoa that may be found in ocular tissue, or in corneal or conjunctival scrapings.

Principle
The acetic acid allows the stain to permeate the cell walls. The nuclei then absorb the chromotrope red dye, showing nuclear details. Nonprotozoal material and debris do not stain and take up only the green dyes.

Procedure
Manufacturer-prepared reagents are readily available. Trichrome stain is stable, can be kept at room temperature, and does not require dilution (Baron et al. 1994). A good stain will appear extremely dark purple. Use only certified dyes. Addition of 1 g extra Chromotrope 2R may be necessary to detect microsporidia. Prepare as follows (Balows et al. 1991):

Chromotrope 2R	6.0 g
Light-green SF	1.5 g
Fast-green FCF	1.5 g
Phosphotungstic acid (CP)	7.0 g
Acetic acid (glacial)	10.0 mL
Distilled water	1000.0 mL

Add the dry chemicals to a large dry flask (approximately 2 liters) and swirl about to mix. Slowly add the acetic acid while mixing with a stirring rod until all of the stain reagents are moistened. Cover completely. Ripen the mixture by allowing to stand approximately 30 minutes. Slowly add the distilled water while mixing, to dissolve stain completely. Store in a stoppered bottle at room temperature.

1. Fix smears in 70% ethanol for 5 minutes.
2. Place in 70% ethanol with addition of iodine (D'Antoni's) for 2 minutes.
3. Place in two changes of 70% ethanol for a duration of 5 minutes, then again for 2 to 5 minutes.
4. Flood smear with trichrome (or place in a staining jar) for 10 minutes.
5. Place in 90% ethanol acidified with 1% acetic acid for a few seconds—no longer.
6. Dip in 100% ethanol.
7. Dip in two changes of absolute alcohol for 2 minutes each.
8. Dip in two changes of xylene for 2 minutes each.
9. Mount in a mounting medium and coverslip.

Interpretation
Amoebic cysts stain red and some detail may be seen. Nuclei and inclusions are red with a tinge of purple. Protozoan trophozoites cytoplasm have a blue-green appearance, and nuclei stain purple to red. Microsporidia stain red, but may

appear very small and elongated (approximately 3.5 to 4 μm in length and 1.5 μm in width). Background and other cells stain green.

Limitations
An old specimen or inadequate fixation may result in organisms staining pale or not at all. Mature cysts need additional fixation and generally do not stain as well as young cysts and spores. Degenerative cysts and spores may not stain and may appear green. White blood cells, yeast, tissue cells, and other cells of human origin may resemble or be mistaken for parasitic organisms in their appearance. Laboratorians must learn to differentiate extraneous materials from actual parasites (Fritsche 1992).

Quality control
Control slides should be run with known positives and one without but containing white cells as in a peripheral blood smear. A file of permanent stained slides of known positives as well as reference photomicrographs should be kept in work area and referred to.

REFERENCES

Balows A, Hausler WJ, Herrmann KL, et al.: Manual of clinical microbiology, 5th Edition. ASM, 1991: 1312.

Baron EJ, Peterson L, Finegold S (eds.): Bailey and Scott's diagnostic microbiology, 9th Edition. St. Louis: C. V. Mosby, 1994, p. 302, 303, 788.

Fritsche TR: Identification aids: Artifacts. In Isenberg (ed.): Clinical microbiology procedures handbook. Volume 2, 7.10.1, Washington, DC: American Society of Microbiology, 1992.

4.1.7. Grocott-Gomori Methenamine Silver (GMS) Stain

Purpose
The incidence of fungal keratitis (keratomycosis) has increased in the last two decades. This has been attributed to the use and abuse of topical corticosteroids, to contact lens wear, and to the use of broad-spectrum antibiotics (Khairallah et al. 1992). Contaminated donor corneas have been implicated in certain cases of fungal keratitis with disastrous consequences. Furthermore, our understanding of fungi has improved, as well as laboratory methods for the diagnosis, and hence the early detection and management, of these infections (Koenig 1986; Taylor and Tabbara 1987).

Principle
To detect positive fungal elements that, once stained, take on a silver or black color. The light green counterstain is used to stain the background a contrasting color. Hematoxylin also may be used.

Preparation
Materials and reagents for the Gomori methenamine silver stain (modified by Forster et al. 1976):

1. Gelatin-coated glass slides (stored at −20°C to 0°C)
2. Chromic acid solution, 5%
3. Methenamine silver nitrate solution:
   Methenamine, 3%.. 100 mL
   Silver nitrate, 0.1% .... 7 mL
4. Gold chloride, 0.1%
5. Sodium thiosulfate solution, 2%
6. Stock light green solution:
   Light green, S.F. .... 0.2 g
   Distilled water.. 100 mL
   Glacial acetic acid .... 0.2 mL
7. Absolute methyl alcohol
8. Distilled water

Procedure
1. Fix slide in absolute methyl alcohol for 5 minutes.
2. Oxidize in 5% chromic acid for 30 minutes.
3. Immerse in preheated methenamine silver nitrate solution for 20 minutes.
4. Wash with six changes of distilled water.
5. Tone for 2 to 4 minutes in 0.1% gold chloride.
6. Rinse with two changes of distilled water.
7. Immerse in 2% sodium thiosulfate solution for 2 minutes.
8. Wash with tap water.
9. Counterstain for 1 minute with fresh 1:5 dilution in distilled water of stock light green solution.
10. Air dry, clean and mount.
11. Examine by light microscopy using 400× and 1000× magnification.

Interpretation
Fungal elements stain silver to black, as shown in Plate 20 of *Aspergillus flavus* and Plate 21 of *Fusarium solani*. Using a low-power objective, fungal elements can easily be seen in a tissue section, as shown in Figure 4.4 along Descemet's membrane. *Acanthamoeba* cell walls stain silver, as depicted in a corneal tissue section in Plate 22. Microsporidia and others stain primarily silver and then only if the cell wall is intact (Davis et al. 1990).

REFERENCES

Davis RM, Font RL, Keisler MS, Shadduck JA: Corneal microsporidiosis: A case report including ultrastructural observations. Ophthalmology 1990; 97(7):954–957.

Forster RK, Wirta MG, Solis M, Rebell G.: Methenamine silver-stained corneal scrapings in keratomycosis. Am J Ophthalmol 1976; 82:261–265.

Khairallah S, Byrne KA, Tabbara KF: Fungal keratitis in Saudi Arabia. Doc Ophthalmol 1992; 79:269–276.

Koenig SB: Fungal keratitis. In Tabbara KF, Hyndiuk RA (ed.): Infections of the eye. Boston: Little, Brown, 1986: 331.

Taylor PB, Tabbara KF: Fungal keratitis. In de Luise VP, Tabbara KF (eds.): Peripheral corneal diseases. Boston: Little, Brown, 1987:44–48.

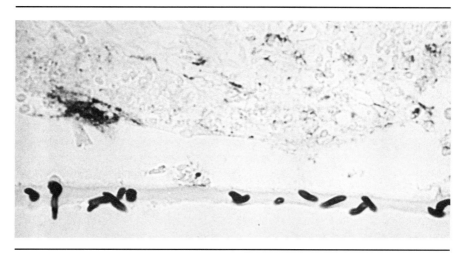

Figure 4.4
Fungal hyphae can easily be seen under low magnification showing hyphae along Descemet's membrane with one projection into the vitreous. GMS stain, 40× magnification.

4.1.8. Hematoxylin and Eosin (H&E) Tissue Stain

Purpose
Trophozoites do not stain by many stains used in parasitology, but are distinguished by their morphology. Other cytologic studies also may require this simple, fast stain for tissue.

Principle
A differential permanent stain that combines basic dye used to stain acidic structures such as nuclear chromatin and acidic eosin dye that reacts with basic substances such as cytoplasmic and cell wall structures.

Procedure
Reagents are readily available by several manufacturers. Using sections cut at approximately 5 mm (Balows et al. 1991), dip in each solution as follows:

1. Two changes of xylol, approximately 2 minutes each
2. Two changes of absolute ethanol, approximately 1 minute each
3. One change of 95% ethanol for 1 minute
4. One change of 90% ethanol for half a minute
5. One change of 80% ethanol for half a minute
6. One change of 60% ethanol for half a minute
7. Two changes of distilled water or until slides appear to run clear
8. Harris hematoxylin combined in glacial acetic acid (5 mL acetic acid and 100 mL hematoxylin) for approximately 2 minutes
9. Rinse slides in distilled water
10. Place in deionized water that has been alkalinized with 20 to 40 drops ammonium hydroxide for approximately 3 seconds (section will immediately appear blue)

11. Rinse in two changes of deionized water to remove the ammonia
12. Counterstain in a picro-eosin solution for about one-half a minute
13. Two changes of 95% ethanol for 1 minute each
14. Two changes of absolute ethanol for 1 minute in the first and 2 minutes in the second rinse
15. Two changes of xylol for approximately 1 minute each
16. Mount in neutral pH mounting fluid.

Interpretation

Cytologic details may be seen in most cells. Red blood cells appear brilliant eosinic orange-red. Morphologic characteristics of parasites such as *Acanthamoeba spp* are readily seen in trophozoite, as shown in Plate 23.

A lower-power objective may be used to scan an area in a tissue section, and cysts can be found deep in the stromal layers of the cornea, as depicted in Plate 24.

Quality control

A tissue slide with normal cytologic characteristics should be run with each patient slide for comparison.

REFERENCE

1. Balows A, Hausler WJ, Herrmann KL, et al.: Manual of clinical microbiology, 5th Edition. ASM, 1991: 1307.

4.1.9. Papanicolaou (PAP) Stain for Demonstrating Intranuclear Inclusions

Purpose

For the demonstration of intranuclear inclusions as seen in herpes simplex, herpes zoster, cytomegalovirus, adenovirus, and measles. Other differential stains may react too strongly with nuclear acids and obliterate these details. Staining characteristics help separate these from other viruses that do not contain nuclear but exhibit only cytoplasmic inclusions (Plotkin et al. 1971).

Principle

The intranuclear mass combines with acidic or anionic dye because of its cationic substances, resulting in a red mass separated by nonstaining chromatin.

Procedure

1. Fix slide immediately in Bouin's solution.
2. Stain in Harris hematoxylin for 30 seconds.
3. Wash in tap water.
4. Differentiate in acid alcohol approximately 2 minutes.
5. Wash in deionized water.
6. A lithium carbonate rinse is used for bluing.
7. Wash in tap water.
8. 50% ethanol, 10 dips.

9. 70% ethanol, 10 dips.
10. 80% ethanol, 10 dips.
11. 95% ethanol, 10 dips.
12. Stain in Orange G, 1 1/2 minutes.
13. Rinse using two changes of 95% ethanol.
14. Stain in EA-50 (Eosin modified) for 30 seconds.
15. Rinse in three changes of 95% ethanol.
16. Rinse in two changes of 100% ethanol.
17. Rinse in 100% ethanol - xylol (1:1) solution for two minutes.
18. Rinse in two changes of xylol.
19. Mount in Permount or other suitable fixative and coverslip.

Interpretation
Inclusions will stain as a red intranuclear mass with a clear halo and marginated chromatin, which appears as a negative halo around the nucleus. Additional morphologic characteristics of cells can be found in Chapter 5: Ocular Cytology.

REFERENCE

1. Plotkin J, Reynaud A, Okumoto M: Cytologic study of herpetic keratitis. Arch Ophthalmol 1971; 85:597–599.

4.1.10. Impression Cytology Staining Procedure

Purpose
For the cytological study of changes in the ocular surface of the eye that may be seen in various disorders, particularly dry eye (Blodi et al. 1988). Topical vitamin A ointment has been shown to reverse the changes and to improve the symptoms and visual acuity in a variety of non–Vitamin-A–deficient causes of conjunctival keratinization and dry eye (Tseng 1985). Vitamin A may be locally deficient because of scar formation and subsequent loss of vascularity (Tseng et al. 1985). Impression cytology is an efficient means of evaluating goblet cell population when establishing the diagnosis of dry eye syndromes (Nelson et al. 1983) and may have a role in monitoring the progress during topical vitamin A therapy.

Principle
Stained filter papers are examined by light microscopy while the integrity of the anatomic location is maintained. The goblet cells take on a brightly stained appearance while epithelial cells stain blue to pink (if keratinized).

Materials
1. Glass staining jars (to accommodate size of staining sample holder).
2. Teflon sample holder (a plastic tissue culture plate may be modified for this use).
3. Precleaned microscope slides.
4. 24 × 60-mm glass coverslip.

Reagents: modified papanacolaou stain (Armed Forces Institute of Pathology 1987)

1. Glacial acetic acid
2. 37% Formaldehyde—
3. 70% Absolute ethyl alcohol
4. 1% Periodic acid

   } Used for fixative

5. Schiff's reagent (keep refrigerated)
6. Sodium metabisulfite
7. Gill's hematoxylin—
8. Scott's tap water substitute
9. 95% Ethanol alcohol
10. Modified orange G
11. Modified eosin Y

    } Used in stain procedure

12. Xylene
13. Permount or suitable mounting medium

Procedure

1. Fill staining jars with 250 mL or more of each reagent listed in Reagents section, numbers 4 through 11. Cover reagents.
2. Perform staining procedure as follows and demonstrated in Figure 4.5:

Solution	Time
a. Rehydrate in 70% ethanol alcohol	2 minutes
b. Tap water rinse	10 dips
c. 1% Periodic acid	2 minutes
d. Tap water rinse	10 dips
e. Schiffs reagent	2 minutes
f. Tap water rinse	10 dips
g. Sodium metabisulfite 0.5%	2 minutes
h. Tap water rinse	10 dips
i. Gill's hematoxylin	2 minutes
j. Tap water rinse	10 dips
k. Scott's tap water substitute	2 minutes
l. Tap water rinse	10 dips
m. Dehydrated in 95% ethyl alcohol	10 dips
n. Modified Orange G	2 minutes
o. 95% ethyl alcohol (2 changes)	3 minutes
p. Modified eosin Y	2 minutes
q. 95% ethyl alcohol (2 changes)	5 minutes
r. Dehydrated in absolute alcohol	2 minutes
s. Transfer to xylene	5 minutes

3. Stained filter papers are then mounted using mounting medium. Each slide will contain three papers (four slides per patient), and a coverslip is affixed.
4. Label slide with identification number, right or left eye, and position numbers.
5. Place slides on a slide tray and allow to remain horizontal.
6. Smears are then examined, taking care not to disturb mounting fluid.

Reading

1. Slides are examined first under 10× to determine areas with greatest goblet cell concentration, cell–cell relationship, etc.

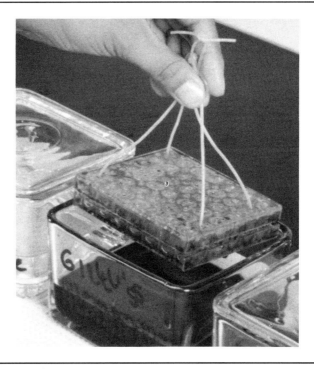

Figure 4.5
A tissue culture plate is modified for staining of filter papers obtained from impression cytology. The plastic or wire handle is tied on, and holes have been made to allow stain to seep through as the tray is taken from jar to jar of stains and washes.

2. Goblet cells, which now stain intensely pink, are viewed and counted under the 40× objective. A differential count is used to approximate the number of Goblet cells per 100 epithelial cells, using a standard differential counter, as demonstrated in Figure 4.3.
3. Morphologic changes in epithelial cells are noted (i.e., enlargement, metachromic changes in cytoplasm, nucleus, etc.).
4. All inflammatory cells present are counted, quantitated per 100 epithelial cells, and reported.
5. A staging system may be used, as defined by Tseng (1985) or Nelson and colleagues (1983), to determine epithelial changes described in detail in Chapter 5: Ocular Cytology.
6. Presence or absence of mucus should also be noted.

Interpretation
Patients with mild scarring of the conjunctiva show a greater number of goblet cells, as seen in Plate 25, whereas patients with severe conjunctival scarring and keratinization show decreased or total absence of the goblet cells by impression cytology, as evident in Plate 26.

REFERENCES

Armed Forces Institute of Pathology: Histological staining procedure manual. Washington, DC: 1987:304–310.

Blodi BA, Byrne KA, Tabbara KF: Goblet cell population among patients with inactive trachoma. Int Ophthalmol J 1988; 12(1):41–45.

Nelson JD, Havener VR, Cameron JD: Cellulose acetate impressions of the ocular surface, dry-eye state. Arch Ophthalmol 1983; 101:1869–1872.

Tseng SCG: Impression cytology and squamous metaplasia. Ophthalmology June 1985; 92:728–733.

Tseng SCG, et al, "Topical Retinoid Treatment for Various Dry-Eye Disorders", Ophthalmology 92: 717–727, June, 1985.

4.2. FLUORESCENCE MICROSCOPY: RAPID AND PERMANENT STAINS

Dyes referred to as "fluors" or "fluorochromes" are called so because of their ability to become excited after exposure and subsequent absorption of ultraviolet light of short wavelength. As these molecules return to their normal state they release these higher energy levels, creating a visible light of a longer wavelength than the light source that excited them. This type of self-illumination is referred to as "fluorescence." Microscopes were developed to exploit this enhanced detection method by employing a light source emitted from above, referred to as "epifluorescence." The light source passes through an excitation filter, which provides the desired wavelength for the particular fluorochrome used, and a special barrier filter prevents this light from hurting the eyes.

Some stains are absorbed directly by a particular organism fluorescing either the entire agent or a property of the object, such as cell walls. By employing the use of a counterstain, the fluorescing object can appear bright against a dark background, depending on the dye used. Knowledge of the affinity certain organisms have for fluorescent dyes allows us to detect these in clinical specimens or to identify morphologic features once obtained in culture. Some stains are used for temporary preparations and others are able to be coverslipped and preserved as a permanent record of the causative agent. A slide film may provide a permanent record and also may be useful to keep a study identification file at the work station. We used a Nikon fluorescence microscope with an FX-35 camera attachment and Kodak Ektachrome 160 Tungsten Professional (EPT-135) slide film for the purpose of building a slide library.

4.2.1. Calcofluor White for the Detection of Fungi and Parasites

Purpose
Calcofluor white stain is a rapid staining procedure used to detect fungi, *Acanthamoeba* cysts, or microsporidia spores in smears from clinical specimens.

Principle
Calcofluor white binds to β1-3, β1-4 polysaccharides such as cellulose, and chitin, and fluoresces bright apple-green when exposed to long-wavelength ultraviolet light or short-wavelength visible light. Cell walls of fungi contain large amounts of chitin, and therefore yeast cells, hyphae, and pseudohyphae are readily visualized. Nonspecific staining of *Acanthamoeba* cysts and spores of microsporidia also have been observed.

Materials
1. Fluorescence microscope
2. Microscope slides and coverslips
3. Calcofluor white stain (Fungi Fluor, Polysciences Inc., Warrington, PA)
4. Absolute methyl alcohol
5. 0.1% Evans blue dye dissolved in distilled water.

Procedure
1. Fix slide in methanol for 3 to 5 minutes.
2. Add several drops of a solution prepared as follows: Combine equal amounts of 0.1% calcofluor white stain and 0.1% Evans blue dissolved in distilled water.
3. After 5 minutes, remove excess stain and apply a coverslip.
4. Examine using a fluorescence microscope for characteristic apple-green (or red if filter is used) chemofluorescence of fungi and amoebic cysts.
5. If permanent slides are desired, periodic acid-Schiff or Grocott-Gomori methenamine silver stains can be done without interference from a slide previously stained with calcofluor white.

Interpretation
1. Positive fluorescence is apple-green (or bright orange-red if filter is used).
2. Background and other cells stain red-brown.

Note: Background fluorescence may be prominent, but fungi exhibit more intense fluorescence, as shown in Plate 27 of *Aspergillus flavus* fungi obtained from culture media.

Cell walls of amoebic cysts and spores of microsporidia cells walls exhibit fluorescence.

Limitations
Immature cell walls of parasites and aging hyphae may lose their ability to hold calcofluor stain in decreasing amounts, as evident in Plate 28, or may not stain at all by this method.

BIBLIOGRAPHY

Hageage GJ, Harrington BJ: Use of calcofluor white in clinical mycology. Lab Med 1984; 15:109–112.

Wilhelmus KR, Osato MS, Font RL: Rapid diagnosis of acanthamoeba using calcofluor white. Arch Ophthalmol 1986; 104:1309–1312.

4.2.2 Potassium Hydroxide–Calcofluor White Procedure

Purpose
The recent increase in immunocompromised patients asssociated with human immunodeficiency virus (HIV) and their susceptibility to opportunistic fungal infections has renewed emphasis for more rapid detection methods to identify these organisms in ocular infections. Arffa et al. (1985) compared the use of calcofluor white alone with the ink-KOH for detecting fungi in ocular specimens from experimentally infected rabbits. Although use of calcofluor alone may be much quicker, the ink-KOH method was more sensitive than calcofluor white alone (Arffa et al. 1985). Other investigators have suggested ways of improving its use (Harrington & Hageage 1991), including that of combining with KOH (potassium hydroxide) for enhanced detection of fungi in clinical specimens.

Principle
Potassium hydroxide in solution with calcofluor white, a fluorescent brightener of textiles, enhances the visualization of fungal elements in microscopic specimens. Calcofluor white binds to both chitin and cellulose in fungal cell walls and fluoresces bright green to blue.

Preparation (Isenberg 1992):
1. 15% potassium hydroxide solution
   Water (distilled) .... 80 mL
   Potassium hydroxide .... 15 g
   Glycerol .... 20 mL
   Dissolve KOH in water and glycerol. Store at 25°C, and re-prepare if a precipitate forms.
2. 0.1% (wt/vol) calcofluor white solution
   Water (distilled) .... 100 mL
   Calcofluor white stain .... 1 g
   (Fungifluor, Cellufluor; Polysciences Co., Warrington, PA, U.S.A.)
   Mix, heating gently, if precipitate develops (or filter if persistent). Store in the dark at room temperature.

Procedure
1. Place specimen on clean glass slide.
2. Add a drop of each solution (15% KOH and calcofluor white).
3. Mix and cover with glass coverslip.
4. Allow to sit at room temperature until material is clear (warming slide will hasten process).
5. Examine using a fluorescence microscope with 10× and 40× to 50× objective or 100× oil.

Interpretation
Fungi stain bright green or blue-white, depending on the filter.

Quality control
1. Before use, check reagents weekly and with each new batch prepared.
2. Use an active culture of *Candida albicans* for a positive control; yeast cell walls stain bright green or blue-white, depending on the UV filter used.
3. A negative control is prepared from straight KOH and calcofluor white solution and should exhibit no fluorescence.

Limitations
Nonspecific fluorescence from human cellular materials and fibers (natural and synthetic) is quite common. Interpretation of the highlighted structures depends on traditional fungal morphologic features and experience of the observer.

REFERENCES

Arffa RC: Calcofluor and ink-potassium hydroxide preparation for identifying fungi. Am J Ophthalmol 1985; 100:719–723.
Harrington BJ, Hageage GJ: Calcofluor white: Tips for improving its use. Clin Microbiol Newsl 1991; 13:3–5.
Isenberg (ed.): Handbook, Clinical Microbiology Procedures, 6.4, Vol. 2. Washington, DC: ASM, 1992.

4.2.3 Acridine Orange Fluorescent Stain

Purpose
For the fluorochromic staining of nucleic acids and may be used for highlighting bacteria in broth media or blood culture.

Principle
The fluorochrome acridine orange binds to nucleic acid by intercalating within the nucleic acid. Initially, this is a viable dye because it fluoresces green if the organism is alive and red if it is not. This is only temporary, however, because the dye process itself does render the organism dead.

Materials
1. Acridine orange stain (BBL, Cockeysville, MD U.S.A or DIFCO, Detroit, MI U.S.A.)
2. Tween 80 (DIFCO Laboratories, Detroit, Michigan)
3. Sodium phosphate, dibasic
4. Citric acid monohydrate
5. Fluorescence microscope

Stock stain solution preparation
1. Acridine orange stain
   a. Acridine orange .... 1.0 g
   b. Tween 80 .... 2.0 mL
   c. Distilled water .... 1000 mL

2. McIlvaine's buffer pH 3.8
   a. Sodium phosphate, dibasic .... 10.081 g
   b. Citric acid monohydrate... 13.554 g
   c. Distilled water... 1000 mL
3. Storage
   a. Store stock stain and McIlvaine's buffer in 10-mL aliquots at −10°C.
   b. Stable for 1 year.

Working stain solution
1. Allow stain and buffer to thaw completely.
2. Withdraw 0.5 mL buffer and mix the remainder with the stock stain.
3. Use the 0.5-mL aliquot of buffer for the mounting medium.

Staining procedure (Brinser 1984)
1. Air dry smear(s).
2. Fix in methyl alcohol for 5 minutes and allow to air dry.
3. Stain for 5 minutes in the working solution of acridine orange stain.
4. Wash gently with distilled water and allow to air dry.
5. Mount using 1 drop of McIlvaine's buffer and coverslip.
6. Examine slides using a fluorescence microscope with the following options:
   a. Darkfield condenser
   b. Exciter filter (BG 12)
   c. Barrier filter (47)
   d. Using a 10× and 40× to 50× objective (100× and 400–500× magnification), search for fluorescing agents and examine morphology with a 100× (1000× magnification) oil immersion objective.

Interpretation
1. DNA takes on a green color.
2. RNA takes on a red or orange color.
3. Bacterial cells will stain red or orange.
4. Fungi will stain either green or red color, as shown in Plate 29 yeast cells.

Quality control
Run a known positive bacterial or fungal smear and a negative control using only buffer mixed with acridine orange working solution. Run control and patient smears at the same time and repeat with fresh reagents if expected results are not achieved.

REFERENCE

Brinser JH: Practical ocular microbiology course 557. Department of Ophthalmology, College of Medicine, University of South Florida, 1984.

4.2.4 Auramine-Rhodamine Fluorochrome Stain

Purpose

All acid-fast agents, including mycobacteria and sporozoan parasites, will stain with auramine or rhodamine or both. The most widely used stain of this type is that of Truant, described in the following procedure. A counterstain is used to prevent nonspecific fluorescence and to stain background a contrasting darker color. It is generally more sensitive and reliable than most acid-fast stains.

Principle

Mycobacteria cell walls are rich in mycolic acid, which has an affinity for auramine and rhodamine fluorochromes. These dyes then bind to the mycobacteria and also many sporozoa, appearing bright yellow or orange against the green background of the counterstain, potassium permanganate.

Reagents

Manufacturer-prepared reagents are widely available from Sigma Chemical Co. (St. Louis, MO) and other chemical supply companies. Working solutions may be prepared as follows:

Stock stain solution

Auramine O	1.5 g
Rhodamine B	0.75 g
Phenol	10.0 mL
Glycerol	75.0 mL
Distilled water	50.0 mL

Mix all of the above and heat until warm, stirring vigorously during the last 5 minutes. Filter through glass wool and pour cooled mixture into a clean glass bottle with a stopper, which may be refrigerated at 4°C and stored for several months.

Decolorizer

Prepare decolorizer by mixing concentrated hydrochloric acid (0.5 mL) with 70% ethanol (100 mL) and store in a glass-stoppered bottle kept at room temperature.

Counterstain

Potassium permanganate	0.5 g
Distilled water	100.0 mL

Mix well and filter through glass wool and store in brown glass-stoppered bottle, this counterstain may be stored at room temperature and is good for at least 6 months.

Procedure
1. Heat fix slide by placing on a slide warmer at 56° to 65°C for 2 hours, or this may be left overnight.
2. Place slide on staining rack and cover smear with stock auramine-rhodamine stain solution, leaving on for 15 minutes at room temperature.
3. Rinse slide gently with distilled water.
4. Decolorize with prepared hydrochloric acid/ethanol for 2 to 3 minutes.
5. Rinse stain off thoroughly with distilled water.
6. Flood slide with counterstain solution of potassium permanganate for 3 minutes.
7. Rinse well with distilled water and allow to air dry.
8. Examine under ultraviolet light source used for fluorescence microscopy with 40× objective and confirm suspect organisms using 100× oil immersion.

Interpretation
Acid-fast organisms stain positively and appear bright yellow-orange against a dark greenish background, as does *Mycobacterium tuberculosis* and other agents, which exhibit varying degrees of fluorescence in the spectrum. Slides may be restained with traditional stains such as Ziehl-Neelsen or Kinyoun if desired for confirmation or to differentiate morphologic features.

Quality control
As with other fluorescence methods, a known positive control should be run along with patient smear and a negative control of reagents only.

BIBLIOGRAPHY

Balows A, Hausler WJ, Herrmann KL, et al.: Manual of clinical microbiology, 5th Edition. Washington, D.C.: American Society for Microbiology, 1991: 1311.
Baron EJ, Peterson L, Finegold SM: Bailey and Scott's diagnostic microbiology, 9th Edition. St. Louis: C. V. Mosby, 1994.
Morse WC: Mycobacter lab methods, Report No. 317. Denver, CO: U.S. Army Medical Research and Nutrition Laboratory, 1992.

4.2.5. Direct Fluorescent Antibody Method for the Detection of *Chlamydia trachomatis*

Direct immunofluorecence using monoclonal antibodies has recently become the gold standard in evaluating "true positives" of *Chlamydia trachomatis* infections. As opposed to a culture positive in which the organism has been grown in cell culture, the sensitivity of this method may detect true clinical cases in which the organism was not viable or failed to grow in cell culture. The performances of a commercial nucleic acid hybridization test (Gen-Probe Pace 2 *Chlamydia trachomatis*) and two commercially available enzyme immunoassays (EIAs) (Abbott Chlamydiazyme and Pharmacia *Chlamydia* EIA) were evaluated against cell culture and Syva Microtrak for the detection of *C. trachomatis* infection at a public health center (Warren et al. 1993). These investigators reported that the sensitivity and specificity for each of these methods positivity rate by true-positive definition as opposed to a culture positive were reported as follows: Gen-Probe, 96.7% and 99.6%; Chlamydiazyme, 77.5% and 100%; Pharmacia EIA, 77% and 100%; cell culture, 80% and 100%. Syva Microtrak and Gen-Probe had identified 12 cases of *C. trachomatis* infection for which culture was negative, concluding that these methods were a good alternative to cell culture for the detection of *C. trachomatis*. These findings support those of Iwen et al. (1991), who in a similar study showed tissue culture to have a sensitivity of 90.3%. Because many laboratories lack the facilities or resources for cell culture studies, alternative nonculture techniques may both be reliable and offer same-day results. However, it is highly recommended that a more satisfactory gold standard for microbiologic assay of these infections would be to use a combination of tests, as suggested by other investigators (Schachter 1991).

Purpose
For the detection of *Chlamydia trachomatis* from clinical specimens or to confirm culture positives by direct fluorescein conjugated monoclonal antibody fluorescence microscopy

Principle
Monoclonal antichlamydial antibodies prepared against the major outer membrane proteins present in all 15 known human serovars of *Chlamydia trachomatis* and in both forms of the organism (i.e., infectious elementary body and the metabolically active reticulate body) are labeled with adsorbed, affinity-purified fluorescein isothiocyanate conjugate. When a specimen is applied directly to the slide well and stained, the antibody conjugate binds specifically to any *C. trachomatis* which may be present in the smear. Any unbound antibody is removed in the rinse step and the stained smears viewed under a fluorescence microscope will detect positive specimens by the fluorescein conjugated monoclonal antibodies exhibiting apple-green fluorescence of elementary or reticulate bodies, contrasted by the reddish orange background of the counterstained cells, as shown in Plate 30.

Specimen collection
Obtain conjunctival scrapings using the procedure described in the section for specimen collection, Conjunctival Scraping Procedure for *Chlamydia* or Cytology Smears. Spread the specimen in both of two wells of a Microtrak slide. Fix with acetone for 10 to 15 minutes and send to the laboratory for staining as soon as possible. These may also be frozen at $-70°C$ until ready to process.

Reagents and materials (Syva Microtrak)
Allow all slides and reagents to come to room temperature before use.

1. Monoclonal antibody solution
2. Fluorescein isothiocyanate conjugate
3. Distilled water
4. Mounting fluid and glass coverslips

Procedure
1. Add 20 μl reagent 1 and 20 μl reagent 2 to each of the fixed specimen and control wells. The entire area of the well must be covered.
2. Place in a well-humidified slide chamber and incubate at room temperature for 15 minutes. Do not allow antibodies to dry onto specimen, because this could cause nonspecific binding.
3. Aspirate the remaining reagent and discard.
4. Rinse the slides gently by agitating in a jar or tray of distilled water 10 seconds.
5. Gently shake off excess water and wick off remaining moisture from the edge of the slide with a paper towel or bibulous paper.
6. Air dry slides, then add a drop of mounting fluid to the center of each slide.
7. Place a coverslip on top of slide and remove all air bubbles.
8. Examine slides immediately after staining or store them in the dark at 2° to 8°C for up to 24 hours before reading, making sure they come to room temperature first.
9. Completely scan the 8-mm well using a suitable fluorescence microscope. It is necessary to use a 400× to 500× magnification for scanning and 1000× oil immersion to examine morphology.

Interpretation
The most common forms in *Chlamydia trachomatis*–positive specimens are extracellular elementary bodies, which will appear as individual pinpoints of medium to bright apple-green fluorescence when scanning at 400× to 500×. Under oil immersion at 1000×, elementary bodies appear evenly fluorescing, smooth-edged, and disc shaped, approximately $1/100$th the size of an intact cell.

The positive control slide may be used as a reference comparison to aid in diagnosis. Other forms of the organism may also be present; however, intact chlamydial inclusions are rarely seen. Some chlamydiae that appear 2 to 3 times the size of an elementary body may stain with a peripheral halo. These represent immature organisms such as reticulate bodies released from a ruptured cell.

Limitations
Particles may fluoresce that are irregularly shaped, differ in size and shape from chlamydial organisms, and often appear yellow, red, or white rather than apple-green. These artifacts, as well as "glassy" fluorescence or a dull olive green, should be disregarded.

Quality control
The positive control slide should show at least ten elementary bodies and a contrasting counterstained background of reddish orange color. The negative control slide should not show fluorescence, and only counterstained cells should be visible. If the positive and negative control slides are indistinguishable, the test is invalid.

REFERENCES

Iwen PC, Blair MH, Woods GL: Comparison of the Gen Probe Pace 2 system, direct fluorescent antibody, and cell culture for detecting *Chlamydia trachomatis* in cervical specimens. Am J Clin Pathol 1991; 95:578–582.

Schachter J: Chapter 105: Chlamydiae. In Balows et al. (ed.): Manual of clinical microbiology, 5th Edition. Washington, DC: American Society of Microbiology, 1991: 1045–1053.

Syva Microtrak for *Chlamydia trachomatis:* Manufacturer's package insert, Palo Alto, CA: Syva Co., 94303-0847.

Warren R, Dwyer B, Plackett M, et al.: Comparative evaluation of detection assays for *Chlamydia trachomatis.* Clin Microbiol June 1993; 31(6):1663 –1666.

4.2.6 Syva Microtrak for Herpes Simplex Virus 1 and 2 (HSV1\HSV2)

Herpes simplex viruses (HSV) are ubiquitous among humans. Once acquired, HSV can remain latent in the regional sensory ganglia, then, when reactivated, move back along the sensory nerves to produce recurrent infections. HSV infections include genital lesions, cold sores, pharyngitis, ocular keratitis, and encephalitis.

The viruses are classified as two biologically distinct serotypes (type 1 or 2) according to their genetic and antigenic composition. Although each type has been associated with a characteristic pattern of infection (oral HSV1 and genital HSV2), in actuality the site of infection is not an accurate predictor of the virus type. In fact, HSV1 is now suspected to cause a significant proportion of primary genital herpesvirus. Both types may infect the eye.

Purpose
Specific diagnosis of HSV infection is required in many cases, particularly infections of neonates, immunocompromised patients (including those with acquired immune deficiency syndrome [AIDS]), and individuals in whom herpes encephalitis is suspected. Typing may have utility in the prognosis of a particular case of herpetic keratitis because it has been reported that the recurrence rate of HSV1 is less than that of HSV2 after treatment. The antiviral activity of chemotherapeutic agents also may differ between the two HSV types, and epidemiologic research is being done on an association of HSV infection with other disease processes and some cancers. Secondary bacterial or fungal infection, especially when topical corticosteroids are used (Khairallah et al. 1992), is also common in patients with ocular herpesvirus. Immunofluorescence techniques can identify these risk groups. Because of the high prevalence of past HSV infections in the general population, many patients who develop malignancy, an immunodeficiency such as AIDS, or diseases that may require immunosuppressive therapy may contract HSV infection or reactivation of a past infection. These symptoms can be severe, locally invasive, and can cause considerable mucocutaneous necrosis, or they can spread to contiguous organs, causing a viremia with dissemination to multiple organs, resulting in meningoencephalitis and coagulopathy (Arvin and Prober 1991).

Principle
Monoclonal antibodies that react specifically with HSV1 or HSV2 are prepared and then labeled with fluorescein isothiocyanate. One of these antibodies reacts with a glycoprotein C complex specific for HSV1 and the other two react only with 140,000- or 38,000-dalton proteins, both of which are specific for HSV2. A fourth monoclonal antibody recognizes an HSV2-specific epitope of a glycoprotein B doublet of 120,000 to 130,000 daltons.

The specimen is applied directly to paired slide wells, of which one has HSV1 reagent applied and the other has HSV2 reagent applied. The antibody conjugates then bind specifically to their respective antigens, if present, and the rinse step removes any unbound antibody. When slides are viewed under fluorescence microscopy, positive fluorescence indicates the viral type, HSV1 or HSV2.

Materials

Supplied by Syva Microtrak manufacturer (Syva Microtrak, 1987) and additional materials that may be necessary:

1. Syva Microtrak slides for HSV1\HSV2 with 8-mm wells
2. Lyophilized reagents for HSV1\HSV2, reconstituted with 2 mL reconstitution diluent
3. HSV1\HSV2 antigen control slides
4. Mounting fluid prepared using phosphate buffer, glycerol, and an agent to retard photobleaching adjusted to pH 7.4 (commercially available)
5. Acetone fixative
6. Distilled water
7. Moist chamber or sterile petri dish
8. Micropipette or automatic pipetting system with disposable pipet tips adjustable to 30 μL
9. Glass coverslips
10. Fluorescence microscope with appropriate filter system for fluorescein isothiocyanate methods

Procedure

1. Specimens (obtained according to specimen collection protocol) are spread onto paired wells of test slides. Distribute equal amounts of material to each well.
2. Allow specimens to air dry completely. Incomplete drying can result in cell loss or disintegration during fixation.
3. Flood smear with 0.5 mL acetone fixative and let the entire quantity evaporate.
4. The smear should be stained as soon as possible, but will keep for up to 3 days. Alternatively, smears may be kept at −70°C for up to 6 weeks, but must not be allowed to thaw and refreeze because this has been known to kill the HSV antigen. Higher temperatures, though freezing, are not sufficient for keeping viral slides or tests.
5. Allow the reagents and all slides to reach room temperature before use.
6. Swirl reagents to mix thoroughly.
7. An HSV1- and an HSV2-positive control slide and a negative control slide must be run with each patient or batch. After staining, these also may serve as a reference for staining reactions.
8. Place 30 μL HSV1 reagent in the left-hand well for each test and control slide(s), then discard pipet tip.
9. Replace with fresh tip and place 30 μL HSV2 reagent in the right-hand well of each slide.

10. Ensure that the entire area of each well is covered and use a spreader stick if necessary, taking care not to make contact with the slide itself.
11. Incubate slides in a well-humidified wet chamber (or sterile petri dish modified by using a damp filter paper and two sticks placed horizontally).
12. Incubate at room temperature for 30 minutes or in a 37°C non-CO_2 incubator for 15 minutes. Optimally, this should be done in a dark area such as a cupboard or closed incubator. Do not allow slides to dry up, because this could cause nonspecific binding.
13. At the end of incubation time, aspirate remaining reagent.
14. Rinse slides in a gentle stream of distilled water for 5 to 10 seconds, aiming at the slide surface but taking care not to direct spray pressure directly onto wells because this could cause cells to wash off.
15. Allow slides to completely air dry.
16. Add 1 drop of mounting fluid to each slide well and place a glass coverslip on top of slide. Remove all air bubbles. Slides must be read immediately after staining or kept in the dark at 2° to 8°C for up to 24 hours.
17. View slides under fluorescence microscopy initially using 400× to 500× magnification and identifying under 1000× magnification.

Interpretation
Scan each well for intact cells displaying fluorescence characteristic of infection with HSV1 or HSV2, as described below.

Cell type: This should be a nonsuperficial epithelial; typically basal or parabasal or a multinucleated giant cell.
Quality of staining: Fluorescent apple-green and granular
Stain distribution: Entire cell; greater concentration at edge

A **positive** diagnosis is made when at least one intact cell is identified according to these criteria. The differentiation between HSV1 and HSV2 is based on the reagent well in which characteristic staining was found (i.e., left-hand well is HSV1 and right-hand well is HSV2). Dual infections, though rare, will show staining in both wells. Typing of isolates obtained from culture are recommended for suspected dual infections. **Negative** results are indicated when both fixed, stained smears are free of characteristic fluorescence. At least twenty intact counterstained nonsuperficial epithelial cells must be visible to assure test validity and sufficient specimen amount. Polymorphonuclear leukocytes or red blood cells may not be included in cell count. If a specimen is inadequate, that is, fewer than twenty intact epithelial cells, obtain a fresh specimen or refer to culture for diagnosis.

Quality control
The positive control slide should exhibit fluorescence as described and also may be used as a reference to guide the viewer to expected results. Therefore, control slides should always be read before the patient slides.

The negative control should not show fluorescence, and only background counterstained cells may be seen.

REFERENCES

Arvin A, Prober CG: Herpes simplex viruses. Chapter 75. In Balows A, et al. (ed.): Manual of clinical microbiology, 5th Edition. Washington DC: American Society of Microbiology, 1991: 822–827.

Khairallah SH, Byrne KA, Tabbara KF: Fungal keratitis in Saudi Arabia. Doc Ophthalmol 1992;79:269–276.

Syva Microtrak HSV1/HSV2 Direct specimen identification typing. Test package insert, Syva Co., Palo Alto, California 94303-0847

4.3. OPTICAL MICROSCOPY METHODS FOR VIEWING UNSTAINED SLIDES: PHASE CONTRAST, DARKFIELD, AND BIREFRINGENCE UNDER POLARIZED LIGHT.

Direct observation of unstained material may provide a fast, inexpensive, and reliable means of identification for certain organisms. This can be achieved through knowledge of the causative organisms that may be identified by alternative types of microscopy and through experience with the use of special microscopic techniques of light and refractive indices. In some cases, viewing an unstained slide is the only accepted method of identification available, and in others it may be used in addition to other microscopies using stained slides. The following techniques are largely dependent on the type of specimen obtained and on acquiring the options necessary to perform them on a standard light (or Kohler) illuminated microscope. In most cases these techniques may be performed on specimens previously stained by other methods because they are not color reliant.

4.3.1. Phase Contrast Microscopy

Purpose

For observation of fungi or parasites in tissue or ocular scrapings, and also may be done on bacterial colonies emulsified in water or saline. This technique is useful in separating fungi and parasites from cellular material and other objects of different densities. With practice, microbiologists can learn to recognize morphologies, motility, and various other characteristics that may aid in the diagnosis and provide early presumptive identification of many ocular pathogens.

Principle

Beams of light pass through the object under examination and are partially deflected by different densities or thicknesses, known as "refractive indices," of the object. These light beams may be deflected again when they impinge on a special objective lens, thereby amplifying brightness when aligning in phase (Finegold and Baron 1986), as when passing through material of uniform refractive index. Concurrently, decreasing in amplitude; visualized as darkness, when out of phase, as happens when it passes through areas of different refractive index. This creates a contrast between the object under examination, be it fungi or amoebic cysts, and the background cells or fluid.

Materials
1. Standard light microscope as used for brightfield microscopy
2. Green filter
3. Phase contrast objective lens
4. Microscopic slides and glass coverslips if necessary
5. Immersion oil (if examining bacteria)

Procedure
1. Slides are prepared from direct smears or tissue sections or, in the case of supernatants and emulsions, a wet preparation that is then coverslipped.
2. Smear is examined directly by phase contrast microscopy for evidence of parasites, fungi, and certain bacterial diseases.
3. Objects of greater densities appear bright and the morphology of fixed smears may show distinctive features, dependent on the varying refractive index of the object.

Interpretation
This is based on the task, that is, the motility of the organism can easily be seen with wet preparations of motile trophozoites. Cysts and spores may be identified and some morphology may be seen, but additional light microscopy methods may be useful in identification. Bacterial wet preparations examined under oil immersion (which is of the same refractive index as glass) achieves enough resolution for the visualization of most species. Fungal hyphae can be detected in tissues or direct smears, as shown in Plate 31 of fungi found in Descemet's membrane, which failed to grow in culture.

REFERENCE

Finegold SM, Baron EJ: Optical methods for laboratory diagnosis of infectious diseases. In Bailey and Scott's diagnostic microbiology, 7th Edition. 1986: 70–71.

4.3.2. Darkfield Microscopy

Certain bacteria are so thin they can not be resolved in direct preparations, even using phase contrast microscopy. These are best viewed by darkfield microscopy, an important means of detecting motility and providing presumptive diagnosis of bacteria, particularly spirochetes. Many methods in immunofluorescence microscopy have negated the need for darkfield in many laboratories. However, the cost of materials and reagents for those methods are not feasible for many laboratories to offer this service. Therefore, darkfield microscopy remains an important part of early diagnosis of these diseases and often the only method used in the detection of spirochetes and treponemes from syphilitic chancres and primary infection of Bejel, which is an endemic syphilis in the Middle East (Tabbara 1990), also called *yaws* in Africa. The ocular manifestations of bejel include uveitis, chorioretinitis, and optic atrophy in the late stages if not detected early in the disease (Tabbara et al. 1989). Mucus patches may be seen associated with skin lesion in the early stages, usually in childhood. Conjunctivitis and keratitis caused by *Treponema pallidum* occurs in the United States and may exhibit a distinct clinical picture (Baron et al. 1994).

Purpose
This method is most often used for the demonstration of motile treponemes, which may be found in the exudate expressed from a primary chancre of syphilis.

Principle
Light is refracted off the surface of an object, which appears brightly lit against a black background. This is achieved by providing light from below, which is then blocked in a central circle so that only light from the outer ring will reach the object at a sharp angle, which scatters this light around the edge of the object. When viewed through an objective, flat objects such as host cells and clear liquid do not refract light and provide a dark background. Oil, having the same refractive index as glass, is used to control the path of light on the top lens of the darkfield condenser.

Procedure
1. Tissue and scrapings may be emulsified in sterile saline or a liquid exudate may be used (if too thick, dilute with saline).
2. Coverslip specimen as a wet preparation.
3. Place a drop of immersion oil on the top lens of the darkfield condenser and slowly raise until the oil comes in contact with the bottom of the slide under examination.
4. Adjust so that the light coming into the condenser is the brightest possible. The condenser height is then adjusted so that the brightest light reflects off the many small particles in the specimen.
5. Place a drop of oil on top of the coverslip and view with oil immersion lens at 1000× magnification.
6. The light from below is blocked in a concentric central circle, allowing light from the outer ring only to reach the organism at a sharp angle.

Interpretation
Motility of the organism as well as some morphology can be detected by darkfield illumination. Treponemes will be long (5–20 μm), tightly coiled, and slender. They are quite slow, rarely spiral, and often bend at the middle.

Quality control
It is a good idea to obtain a scraping from the inside of one's cheek to set the lighting for darkfield before receiving the slide. Because there are many nontreponemal spirochetes that inhabit the mouth, this may also provide a visual control or reference for spirochetes if obtained in scraping. Therefore, material for test should NOT be obtained from oral lesions, to avoid reporting of false positive.

REFERENCES

Baron EJ, Peterson LR, Finegold SM: Infections of the head and neck, Chapter 23, In Bailey and Scott's diagnostic microbiology, 9th Edition, 1994; 297–298.

Tabbara KF: Endemic syphilis (bejel). Int Ophthalmol J 1990; 14:379–381.

Tabbara KF, Al Kaff A, Fadel T: Ocular manifestations of endemic syphilis (bejel). Ophthalmology 1989; 96(7):1087–1091.

4.3.3. Polarized Light Microscopy: For the Demonstration of Birefringence

Birefringent hemozoin, which is a component of malarial pigment, can easily detect the presence of any of the four species of malaria (*Plasmodium flaciparum, P. ovale, P. vivax*, and *P. malariae*), but it is not possible to distinguish among the species by this method. The inclusive term *malarial pigment* has been divided into two components, malarial pigment and hemozoin. Hemozoin is a complex crystalline polymer formed from heme incidental to hemoglobin digestion within the digestive vacuoles of replicating trophozoites and schizonts within host erythrocytes. Birefringent hemozoin polymers were observed within the retinal and uveal microcirculation and also in the epibulbar hemorrhage that involved the bulbar conjunctiva by Hidayat et al. (1993). These investigators stressed the fact that traveler's malaria constitutes a large percentage of the 300 million cases of malaria worldwide and may result in death caused by drug resistance and delayed diagnosis.

Purpose
The histopathologic diagnosis of malarial parasitemia of the ocular tissue can be made using polarized light microscopy to demonstrate birefringence of the hemozoin component of malarial pigment.

Principle
Under polarized microscopy, the hemozoin polymer produces birefringence, appearing brightly lit as a starry sky, first reported by Schaudinn in 1903 and more recently regarded as diagnostic of malaria (Lawrence and Olson 1986).

Procedure
1. Thin tissue sections may be prepared without staining or a previously stained smear or tissue may be used without affecting this method.
2. A polarized light system option is used on a standard light microscope.
3. The slide may be scanned under a low-power 100× magnification and closely observed for morphology at 400× to 500× high power. A blue filter may be used to increase contrast.

Interpretation
Under polarized light, the cells and background appear dark, creating a contrast to the brightly appearing crystalline polymers of hemozoin malarial pigment, as shown in Plate 10 tissue.

REFERENCES

Hidayat AA, Nalbandian RM, Sammons DW, et al.: The diagnostic histopathologic features of ocular malaria. Ophthalmology 1993;100(8):1183–1186.

Lawrence C, Olson JA: Birefringent hemozoin identifies malaria. Am J Clin Pathol 1986; 86:360–363.

4.4 ELECTRON MICROSCOPY

There are two types of electron microscopy (EM) used in the laboratory: scanning and transmission. Because the purpose of diagnostic EM is to differentiate and substantiate by observing ultrastructural details, this section deals with preparation and processing of transmission electron microscopy.

4.4.1. Processing Samples for Transmission Electron Microscopy

Because the electron microscope uses differences in electron density of the object to create images, specimen preparation is unlike that used in brightfield microscopy described previously. Using a beam of electrons as the source of illumination, the wavelength is much shorter than UV light and decreases the resolution from 0.2 μm in the light microscope to 0.005 μm in an electron microscope. Along with a major advantage in resolution of the object being examined, there is a disadvantage in that the fixing and preparation process may create artifacts and certain types of specimens are difficult to assess. Examination of the ultrastructural components of cells and organisms found in ocular infections may identify those that are unculturable and may provide a presumptive or definitive diagnosis in many cases. Therefore, the microbiologist and ophthalmologist should become familiar with the fixation and preparation of specimens for EM even when these tests may be sent out for evaluation in another laboratory. Proper fixation is crucial to the quality of this examination.

Purpose
Certain parasites such as Microsporidia (including *Encephalitozoon, Nosema connori,* and *Nosema corneum*) can be found in the conjunctiva and corneas of patients who may be immune compromised or suffering from HIV. Several clinical patterns of microsporidial infection have emerged in AIDS with extensive involvement, including punctate epithelial keratopathy, conjunctival injection, and dissemination involving urinary, respiratory, and ocular tissues (Diesenhouse et al. 1993; Shadduck et al. 1990). Isolated cases of corneal microsporidiosis have also occurred in otherwise healthy patients with no history of ocular disease. Electron microscopy is used to identify to the species level and may be the only method for differentiation of nonculturable or difficult to culture microsporidial and amoebic (*Acanthamoeba, Naegleria*) parasitemias. Other organisms and cells also may benefit from electron microscopy because the ultrastructural components of cells and observance of intracellular bacteria or viruses may indicate a specific disease process.

Principle

An illumination source composed of a tungsten filament heated in a vacuum emitting electrons uses magnetic coils to direct the electron beam that passes through the specimen. The focused electron beam passes through an object the way light passes through a specimen in light microscopy. The dense areas absorb and retard the beam and the less-thick areas are unmodified. Through a series of magnetic coils that refocus and magnify, the image is finally able to be observed visually and transferred to film, resulting in a two-dimensional image of the object.

Procedure

There are three ways one can prepare specimens for transmission electron microscopy (Chapin-Robertson and Edberg 1991):

1. Negatively stain the specimen, whereby the background is stained with a heavy metal such as gold or uranium, which leaves the target object free of the metal, creating a contrast when the microbe or cell appears light while the background appears dark.
2. Freeze etching, whereby the specimen is supercooled, resulting in fractures along the planes within the specimen, which separate by physical impact.
3. Thin sectioning techniques in which the specimen is treated with a fixative such as osmium tetroxide or glutaraldehyde, put through a process of dehydration, and finally impregnated with epoxy resins then sectioned as thin as 0.03 to 0.05 μm and processed by treatment with heavy metals to increase the contrast.

4.4.2. Rapid Fixation Method for Electron Microscopy

The investigation of ultrastructure is crucial to ocular anatomy studies as well as diagnostic histopathology of ocular disease. The following procedure (Shoukrey et al. 1987 and 1991; Shoukrey and Tabbara 1993) reduces the fixation time down to 20 to 40 minutes, thereby limiting the risk of damage to ocular tissue from overfixation and prolonged exposure to dehydrants, which may cause cell shrinkage and lipid extraction. This is especially important when dealing with a hollow soft tissue structure like the eye. This method has demonstrated new subcellular features of ocular tissue for the first time and improved visualization in most tissues of the eye.

Purpose

This rapid one-step method for fixing ocular tissue for electron microscopy may be used for any animal tissue type where both rapid processing and improved visualization is desired.

Principle

The addition of mannose to the mixed glutaraldehyde and osmium tetroxide (OsO_4) fixative slows down the interaction between glutaraldehyde and OsO_4 to give improved more consistent rapid fixation of ocular tissue for EM. Continuity of plasma membranes is well preserved and artifactual blisters are not observed.

Procedure
Prepare the fixative immediately before use as follows:

1. The optimum stabilized fixative consists of 9.75 mol/L sodium cacodylate, 30 mol/L NaCl, 0.1 mol/L mannose, 4 mmol/L $MgCl_2$, 4 mmol/L KCl, 2 mmol/L KH_2PO_4, 1.5% glutaraldehyde, 1 mmol/L $CaCl_2$, and 0.5% OsO_4.
2. Adjust pH to between 7.55 and 7.65 with 1 N HCl before the final addition of OsO_4.
3. Pieces of tissue are immersed in the glutaraldehyde mannose osmium tetroxide fixative while gently agitating for 20 minutes for conjunctiva and 40 minutes for corneal tissue.
4. Briefly rinse tissue fragments in distilled water.
5. Dehydrate through graded concentrations of ethanol.
6. Embed in Epon 812 over propylene oxide.
7. After polymerization, cut blocks on a microtome with a diamond knife.
8. Pick up silver sections on 200-mesh grids.
9. Double stain in uranyl acetate (20 minutes) and lead citrate (5 minutes).
10. View sections and micrograph in an electron microscope (Foreign) at accelerated voltages of 60 and 80 KV.

Interpretation
Membrane tissues of ocular tissue should be well fixed and sharply defined at low magnification. Cysts and other organisms should show clear details of ultrastructural components and nuclei, etc. Microsporidia in keratoplasty specimens may show extracellular spores, viable or nonviable forms with degenerated structures having a vacuolated appearance and surrounded by a thick capsule. Mature spores of *Nosema spp* are surrounded by a thickened translucent cell wall, may have diplokarya, and a polar tubule with five to six coils (Davis et al. 1990). Occurrence of bacterial endosymbionts in *Acanthamoeba spp* trophozoites observed by EM in Figure 4.6. have demonstrated septum formation and bacterial rod binary fission suggesting intracellular multiplication. This characteristic may contribute to increased virulence of these species in corneal keratitis (Fritsche et al. 1993).

Note to the reader:
After electron micrographs are produced the clinician and microbiologist may view the ultrastructural components of parasites and compare with reference isolates previously reported. Pathologist evaluation is often desired and necessary when determining ultrastructure of certain cells. Spores of Microsporidia demonstrate multiple stages of development and polar tubule apparatus can easily be seen, however, other texts in parasitology should be consulted should the microbiologist need additional information for identification of these emerging pathogens. Mitochondrial DNA fingerprinting of *Acanthamoeba* spp may be useful in determining specific taxonomic relationships of members of the genus and suggests that development of specific gene probes is possible (Gautom et al. 1994).

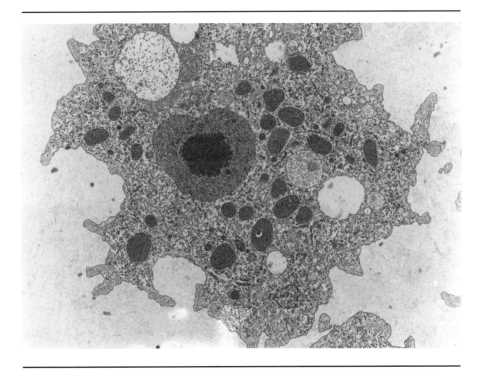

Figure 4.6
Electron micrograph of Acanthamoeba spp *isolated from the cornea. Courtesy of Ro-mesh K. Gautom, Ph.D., Department of Laboratory Medicine, University of Wash-ington, Seattle, Washington.*

REFERENCES

Chapin-Robertson, Edberg SC: Microscopy. Chapter 4. In Balows A, Hausler WJ, Herrmann KL, et al. (eds.): Manual of clinical microbiology, 5th Edition. 1991: 33–34.

Davis RM, Font RL, Keisler MS, Shadduck JA: Corneal microsporidiosis: A case report including ultrastructural observations. Ophthalmology 1990; 97(7):953–957.

Schwartz DA, Govinda GS, Visvesvara GS et al.: Pathologic features and immunofluo-rescent antibody demonstration of ocular microsporidiosis (*Encephalitozoon hellem*) in seven patients with AIDS. Am J Ophthalmol 1993; 115:285–292.

Fritsche TR, Gautom RK, Seyedirashti S, et al.: Occurrence of endosymbionts in *Acan-thamoeba spp* isolated from corneal and environmental specimens and contact lenses. J Clin Microbiol 1993; 31(5):2211–1126.

Gautom RK, Lory S, Seyedirashti S, et al.: Mitochondrial DNA fingerprinting of *Acan-thamoeba spp* isolated from clinical and environmental sources. J Clin Microbiol 1994, 32(4):1070–1073.

Shadduck JA, Meccoli RA, Davis R, Font RL: Isolation of a Microsporidian from a hu-man patient. J Infect Dis 1990; 162:773–776.

Shoukrey NM, Tabbara KF: Ultrastructural study of a corneal keloid. Eye 1993; 7:379–387.

Shoukrey NM, Tabbara KF, Alvarez H: Rapid one step method for fixing ocular tissue of rabbit for electron microscopy (Abstract). ARVO, Invest Ophthalmol Vis Sci 1987; 28(3):24.

Shoukrey NM, Tabbara KF, Alvarez H: Rapid one step method for fixing ocular tissue of rabbit for electron microscopy. Saudi J Ophthalmol 1991; 5(1):50–60.

Ocular Cytology

5

5.1 INTERPRETATION OF GIEMSA STAINED SMEARS

Purpose

The examination of cells from conjunctival scrapings or exudates may provide useful information in making or confirming the diagnosis in many ocular diseases. The presence or predominance of certain types of inflammatory cells or changes in epithelial cells often indicate a specific disease state.

Principle

Giemsa stain is a neutral dye composed of an acidic dye and a basic dye together in the same solution. The colored anion and the colored cation combine to form a colored salt. The salt reacts with and stains certain cell structures purple, the acid component stains other cell ctructures red, and the basic component stains additional cell structures blue.

Interpretation

Normal epithelial cells   Normal conjunctival epithelial cells are of the stratified columnar type (somewhat elongated) and measure 15 to 25 μm in diameter. They have large, round, slightly eccentrally located nuclei that often contain prominent nucleoli (Plate 32). The light basophilic cytoplasm is abundant and slightly granular. Epithelial cells from scrapings of normal conjunctiva come off in sheets and contain nuclei that are uniform in size and staining characteristics.

The normal conjunctiva may show a mild lymphocytosis and may also contain a few polymorphonuclear leukocytes (PMNs). Increased numbers of these cell types may be seen (without a predominance of either) in normal asymptomatic soft (but not hard) contact lens wearers.

Keratinized epithelial cells   In some cases the epithelial cells show degenerative changes. These cells have nuclei that are variable in size, usually larger than normal, and stain irregularly and less intensely. The cytoplasm also shows degenerative changes. Early or partial keratinization is identified by the presence of faint red granules in the cytoplasm as well as a change in the color of the cytoplasm to pinkish (Plate 33). This may progress in certain conditions to complete keratinization, which is characterized by loss of the nucleus and a pink-staining cytoplasm. Normal conjunctival epithelial cells never show keratinization while the epithelial cells of the lid margins are keratinized. Keratinizing and keratinized epithelial cells may occur in exposure of the conjunctiva with ectropion of the eyelid, severe cicatrization as in pemphigoid, trachoma, erythema multiforme, keratoconjunctivitis sicca, and other forms of membranous and pseudomembranous conjunctivitis. Keratinized cells are also seen in vitamin A deficiency and superior limbic keratoconjunctivitis as well as in epithelial plaques and Bitot spots.

Neoplasia.   In neoplastic processes, the epithelial cells may take on bizarre polymorphic and pleomorphic appearances (Plate 34). In neoplasia, nuclear changes are most important. The nucleus is usually bigger, irregular in shape, and may stain darker or lighter than normal. Multiple nucleoli may be present and are often larger than normal. The nucleus:cytoplasm ratio is less (1:1 compared with 1:4–1:6 in normal epithelial cells). The cytoplasm may stain darker blue in many tumors because of increased RNA content.

Multinucleated epithelial cells.   Multinucleated epithelial cells are most commonly known as giant cells, but also may be called polykaryocytes. In the conjunctiva, they usually result from failure of cellular division. As the name suggests, they are much larger than normal epithelial cells and contain several nuclei (Plate 35). Giant cells may be seen in scrapings from patients with herpes simplex, varicella-zoster, cytomegalovirus, measles, Newcastle disease, and trachoma. Tumor cells that are multinucleated are usually very large, irregularly shaped, have scanty cytoplasm and an aberrant chromatin pattern. The nuclei contain enlarged nucleoli—usually four or more. Degenerative changes (vacuolization) of the nucleus and cytoplasm are also seen. Giant cells also may be seen in patients after irradiation; however, these have no characteristic appearance and are extremely variable.

Goblet cells.   Goblet cells may be found in scrapings taken from normal conjunctiva if the scraping is taken from the nasal or temporal conjunctiva and includes the edge of the tarsus. Goblet cells are a special type of epithelial cell with a large clump of clear or pale pink-staining mucoid material contained in a secretory vacuole that has displaced the cytoplasm and pushed the nucleus to the extreme edge of the cell, giving it a half-moon or crescentic shape (Plate 36). Goblet cells are increased in number and are found in atypical distribution in some types of chronic conjunctivitis, including early keratoconjunctivitis sicca and rosacea blepharoconjunctivitis. Other surface disorders such as Stevens-Johnson syndrome and ocular cicatricial pemphigoid may have decreased goblet cell counts.

Inclusion Bodies
Chlamydial. Ophthalmia neonatorum, adult inclusion conjunctivitis, and trachoma (Plate 37) are the *Chlamydia* infections found in the eye. The intracytoplasmic, basophilic inclusion bodies (Halberstaedter-Prowazek bodies) typically associated with *Chlamydia* infections are found much less frequently in scrapings from adults, but may be present in large numbers in scrapings from neonates with inclusion conjunctivitis. *Chlamydia* inclusions are found in the cytoplasm of epithelial cells, although PMNs may contain elementary bodies from phagocytosis. Inclusion bodies in cases of psittacosis may be seen in mononuclear cells. The infected epithelial cells are often swollen and separated from the normal epithelial cells and may show some degenerative cytoplasmic vacuolization. *Chlamydia* inclusions may be seen in any stage of their developmental cycle. Elementary bodies are small (approximately 300 nm in diameter) round structures that take on a reddish-blue or purple (DNA) stain with Giemsa. They are best demonstrated in conjunctival scrapings using fluorescein-conjugated monoclonal antibodies. Once inside the host epithelial cell, elementary bodies differentiate into a blue (RNA) staining, round, oval or bacillary-shaped structure approximately 1 µm long, known as an initial or reticulate body. The initial body divides by binary fission, eventually producing many elementary bodies within the intracytoplasmic inclusion. This aggregate of elementary bodies is typically located near the nucleus, forming a "cap," and is enveloped in a glycogen-rich matrix that stains brown with Lugol's iodine (Plate 38). Iodine staining is not seen with *C. psittaci* inclusions. For diagnostic purposes, when inclusion bodies are not found, but there are numerous PMNs, separation and enlargement of the epithelial cells, lymphocytes, plasma cells, and macrophages, the cytology is suggestive of *Chlamydia* infection. Blast cells and Leber cells also may be seen.
Viral. Viral inclusion bodies may be either eosinophilic or basophilic (Table 5.1). Intracytoplasmic inclusion bodies are typically formed by the large viruses such as vaccinia and variola, whereas intranuclear inclusions are formed by smaller viruses (herpes simplex virus, adenovirus, measles virus, cytomegalovirus, and smallpox virus) (Plate 39). Measles virus, cytomegalovirus, and smallpox virus can produce both intranuclear and intracytoplasmic inclusion bodies.

Pseudoinclusions.   Occasionally one may see any of several types of intracytoplasmic particles (pseudoinclusions) that may resemble *Chlamydia* inclusions and may cause confusion when examining Giemsa-stained scrapings. These include pigment (melanin) granules (Plate 40), phagocytosed debris, nuclear extrusions, free eosinophilic granules, keratin granules, and bacteria. The most common pigment granules are melanin granules that stain black or blue-black or green-blue and can "cap" the nucleus but are usually found scattered throughout the cytoplasm and are present in most of the epithelial cells in the smear. Pigment granules in epithelial cells are a normal finding in scrapings from patients with darkly pigmented skin. Pigment granules are also charac-

Table 5.1
Virus-Induced Inclusion Bodies

Virus	Nuclear	Inclusion bodies cytoplasmic
Herpes simplex	+ (E)	−
Varicella zoster	+ (E)	−
Cytomegalovirus	+ (E)	+ (B)
Adenovirus	+ (E—early) (B—late)	−
Measles	+	+ (E)
Vaccinia	−	+ (E)
Variola	−	+ (E)
Molluscum contagiosum	−	+ (E)
Newcastle disease	−	+ (E)
Rabies	−	+ (E)

E = eosinophilic; B = basophilic.

teristically seen in scrapings from patients with melanoma. Cytoplasmic "blue bodies," which are deep blue-staining lipid-containing phagolysosomes have been described in association with staphylococcal hypersensitivity or topical drug hypersensitivity or toxicity reactions, particularly with neomycin. Scrapings from cases of toxic conjunctivitis also may reveal mononuclear cells, occasional PMN, and mild keratinization of epithelial cells. Eosinophils will be found only if there is an allergic reaction as well.

Polymorphonuclear Leukocytes (PMNs)   PMNs (also known as neutrophils) are round cells, 10 to 12 μm in diameter, easily recognized by their nucleus, which is separated into lobes connected by a narrow filament (Figure 5.1). The cytoplasm stains light pink and contains very small granules that stain light pink to blue-black. PMNs are phagocytic cells, and a PMN response is the reaction seen in all bacterial infections and fungal infections. When large numbers of PMNs are present, the slide should be examined using the oil immersion microscope objective for the presence of bacteria or fungi. Note that all bacteria stain blue with Giemsa. Yeast cells and some of the internal cytoplasmic contents of filamentous fungi stain blue, and the cell walls and septations do not stain. A mucus or fibrinous exudate and cellular debris also may be seen. PMNs are also the predominant cell type in a mixed inflammatory response seen in *Chlamydia* infections, Reiter's disease, psoriasis, and erythema multiforme. It is important to note that corneal damage will always elicit a PMN response, even when caused by a viral infection.

Mononuclear cells
Lymphocytes. Lymphocytes are round or oval cells and may be large (approximately 10 μm in diameter) or small (approximately 7 μm) (Plate 41). The nucleus occupies most of the cell and is spherical, sometimes with slight

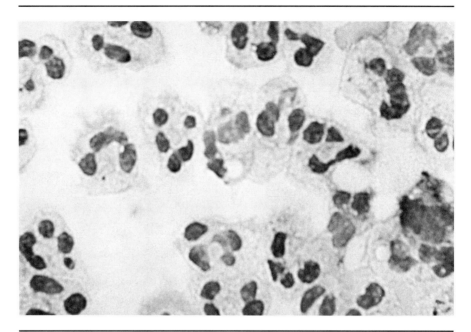

Figure 5.1
A Giemsa-stained conjunctival scraping showing several polymorphonuclear neu-trophils, which are small cells with multilobed nuclei. They are typically indicative of bacterial infection, and the smear should be examined under oil immersion for the presence of bacteria.

indentations. The chromatin stains dark purple and may be clumped, resulting in patches staining a less intense purple. The nucleus is usually somewhat ec-centrically located and is surrounded by a halo of light blue-staining cytoplasm. Lymphocytes are the effectors of the immunologic defenses of the body and ac-complish this by virtue of their ability to generate cells that produce antibody, interferon, and lymphokines, and are also the cells that participate in cell-mediated immune responses.

Monocytes. Monocytes are large cells, 9 to 25 μm in diameter, and are distin-guished from lymphocytes by the large amount of cytoplasm in relation to the size of the nucleus. The nucleus is usually indented and contains loose chro-matin. Monocytes are circulating phagocytic cells and, in local inflammatory reactions, monocytes migrate into the tissue and transform into macrophages.

Mononuclear cells are the predominant cells seen in viral conjunctivitis. Lymphocytes are typically seen in greater numbers than monocytes. These cells may be seen in large numbers in chronic conjunctivitis, but PMNs may be the predominant cell type in early disease. PMNs also may predominate in viral dis-eases if there is corneal necrosis, secondary bacterial infection, or membrane or pseudomembrane formation. In endophthalmitis, the presence of lymphocytes in the aqueous or vitreous indicates either an allergic or parasitic infection.

Mitotic figures.   Lymphocytes may occasionally be seen in any of the various stages of cell division (Plate 42). Although this finding has been attributed to cases of trachoma, it is indicative of active inflammation and may be seen in other cases as well.

Blast cells   Blast cells (immunoblasts, lymphoblasts) result when lymphocytes are exposed to the antigen to which they have been sensitized. These lymphocytes differentiate into blast cells and proliferate; thus blast cells are the precursors of plasma cells (if differentiated from B lymphocytes) or activated T lymphocytes (if differentiated from T lymphocytes). B lymphoblasts have the same structural features as T lymphoblasts and are characterized by enlarged size (15–30 μm diameter), basophilic cytoplasm (due to high RNA content) with vacuoles and lysozomes (Plate 43). There is dispersion of the nuclear chromatin, resulting in a light staining nucleus with a thin marginal layer of heterochromatin. Large nucleoli are often seen. Blast cells may be seen in conjunctival scrapings from any inflammation, especially if acute in nature.

Plasma cells   Plasma cells are highly differentiated B lymphocytes that are responsible for the production of antibodies that participate in the body's humoral defenses against antigens. They are 6 to 20 μm in diameter, may be round, oval, or polyhedral, and have smooth margins (Plate 43). They have a small nucleus that is located at the edge of the cell. The nucleus is rough in appearance because of radially arranged heterochromatin, which produces the characteristic "cartwheel" or "clockface" appearance. The abundant cytoplasm stains dark blue, presumably because of the large amount of RNA needed for the process of protein synthesis. A clear area may be seen adjacent to the nucleus, which is the site of the Golgi apparatus. Plasma cells are never very numerous in conjunctival scrapings and are characteristically seen along with PMNs, lymphocytes, and Leber cells in trachoma, but may be seen in other conditions as well.

Eosinophils   Eosinophils are about the same size and shape as PMNs and typically have bilobed and occasionally mononuclear or trilobed nuclei. Their distinguishing characteristic is the presence of large spherical granules that stain red with Giemsa (Plate 44). Eosinophils are attracted by products released from T lymphocytes, mast cells, and basophils. They release the enzymes such as histaminase, kininase, and aryl sulphatase contained in their granules, which inactivate the vasoactive amines released by mast cells. The net effect of eosinophil activity is to mitigate the allergic inflammatory response and aid in destruction of certain organisms such as parasites. Eosinophils are the predominant cell type seen in acute and chronic vernal and atopic allergic inflammation. A few eosinophils may be seen in contact allergic conjunctivitis caused by cosmetics, medications, or chemical or vegetable irritants, with the exception of some conditions such as pilocarpine sensitivity, which do not elicit an eosinophil response. It should be noted that allergy-induced systemic eosinophilia does not always elicit concomitant conjunctival eosinophilia. Eosinophils are commonly seen along with basophils and mast cells in giant papillary conjunctivitis and along with mononuclear cells, PMNs, and mast cells in ligneous conjunctivitis.

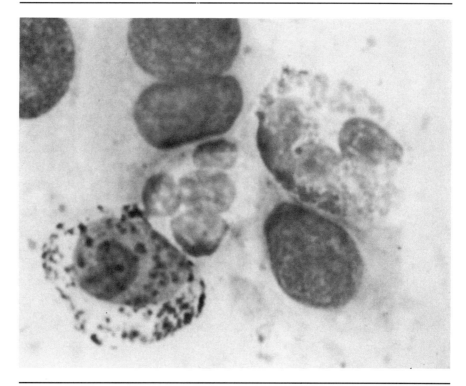

Figure 5.2
A basophil (lower cell) with blue intracytoplasmic granules is seen in a scraping from a patient with allergic conjunctivitis along with a polymorphonuclear neutrophil (middle) and eosinophil (top). Giemsa stain.

Eosinophils also may be seen in the late stages of ocular cicatricial pemphigoid and in parasitic ocular infiltrations. Eosinophilic granules are produced by fragmentation of the cells and are suggestive of vernal conjunctivitis, both the active and the quiescent stages.

Basophils   Basophils are also about the size and shape of PMNs and have indented, bilobed, or multilobed nuclei. The metachromatic cytoplasmic granules stain dark blue and are unevenly distributed and often overlie the nucleus (Figure 5.2). The granules contain histamine, heparin, and the other acid mucopolysaccharides found in mast cell granules. They have IgE surface receptors and have activities similar to mast cells, but are circulating cells rather than tissue fixed. Basophils are never seen in large numbers, but may be associated with eosinophils in allergic inflammation.

Mast cells   Mast cells are the tissue equivalent of basophils and are present in normal subcutaneous and submucosal tissues and may be seen in giant papillary conjunctivitis and ligneous conjunctivitis, vernal conjunctivitis and allergic inflammations, but are rarely seen in conjunctival scrapings from other conditions. They are oval or polyhedral in shape and have a round nucleus that is relatively small in relation to the amount of cytoplasm. The cytoplasm is filled with small, metachromatic granules that stain deep purplish-red with Giemsa. Mast cell granules contain histamine, heparin, and other vasoactive amines. These inflammatory mediators are released on degranulation initiated by combination of their surface IgE with an appropriate antigen.

Leber cells   Leber cells are very large macrophages that are several times the size of an epithelial cell and contain phagocytosed debris that is mainly nuclear in origin (Plate 45). The cytoplasmic border is often not well defined. Leber cells are often found in cases of trachoma, but can also be seen in other kinds of conjunctivitis.

Acanthamoeba *cysts*   The walls of *Acanthamoeba* cysts stain dark blue with Giemsa and the cytoplasm stains light blue to grey. In suspected *Acanthamoeba* keratitis, a trichrome stain may be useful because the trophozoites may be difficult to distinguish from inflammatory cells in Giemsa stained smears. The irregular cell border, vacuolated cytoplasm, and nuclear karyosome are distinctive features demonstrated by the Giemsa technique. It is recommended that questionable smears be stained using calcofluor white or a specific fluorescent antibody stain for positive identification.

Complications

Ideal staining results may not be obtained if the stain components are of poor quality or if the staining procedure is not performed properly. If the stain is alkaline, the pH of the buffered water is not neutral, the smear is thick or overstained, the following abnormal staining characteristics may be seen. Red blood cells appear green or blue. The cytoplasm of cells is light and the cell border is poorly defined. The nuclear chromatin is deep blue to black. The cytoplasmic granules in PMNs, which usually stain very faintly, are deeply overstained, large, and prominent. The granules in eosinophils are blue or gray rather than red.

   In contrast, if the stain is acidic, the pH of the buffered water is acidic, or the smear is understained, the following abnormal staining characteristics may be observed: Red blood cells appear bright red or orange. Nuclear chromatin stains pale blue. The granules in eosinophils stain very intense red.

Significance

The significance of the predominance of various inflammatory cells and other findings in Giemsa stained conjunctival scrapings is summarized below. We estimate the intensity of the cellular response by counting the number of inflammatory cells per 100 epithelial cells. Acute bacterial conjunctivitis generally produces more than 100 polymorphonuclear leukocytes per 100 epithelial cells. Herpes simplex and adenoviral conjunctivitis typically produce less than 100 lymphocytes and monocytes per 100 epithelial cells. Determination of the predominant type of inflammatory cell is simplified by performing a differential count, as for a peripheral blood smear.

Findings	Significance
Predominantly PMNs	Bacterial conjunctivitis
	Chemical conjunctivitis
	Erythema multiforme
	Reiter's syndrome
	Membranes/pseudomembranes
Predominantly lymphocytes	Viral conjunctivitis
	Toxic conjunctivitis
	Allergic conjunctivitis
Mixed PMNs, lymphocytes, monocytes, plasma cells, multinucleated epithelial cells, separated epithelial cells	Presumed *Chlamydia* conjunctivitis
Above findings plus basophilic intracytoplasmic inclusion bodies within epithelial cells	Definite *Chlamydia* conjunctivitis
Eosinophils (with or without free eosinophilic granules)	Allergic conjunctivitis
	Vernal conjunctivitis
	Atopic disease
	Erythema multiforme
	Benign mucous membrane pemphigoid
	Parasitic ocular infections
	Giant papillary conjunctivitis
	Ligneous conjunctivitis
Keratinizing epithelial cells	Keratoconjunctivitis sicca
	Xerophthalmia
	Superior limbic keratoconjunctivitis
	Cicatrization in pemphigoid
	Erythema multiforme
	Epithelial plaques
	Bitot spots
	Membranous and pseudomembranous conjunctivitis
	Some forms of chronic conjunctivitis

Goblet cells   Increased in number and
                                        atypical distribution in:
                                        Keratoconjunctivitis
                                            sicca
                                        Chronic conjunctivitis
                                        Rosacea conjunctivitis
                                        Decreased in number in:
                                        Stevens-Johnson disease,
                                        Cicatricial pemphigoid

REFERENCES

Allansmith MR, Korb DR, Greiner JV: Giant papillary conjunctivitis by hard or soft contact lens wear: Quantitative histology. Ophthalmology 1978;85:766–778.

Hirji NK, Scott J, Sabell AG: Conjunctival cytology in hard and soft contact lens wear. Ophthalmol Physiol Optometry 1985;5:333.

Jones DB, Liesegang TJ, Robinson NM: Laboratory diagnosis of ocular infections. In Cumitech 13, Cumulative techniques and procedures in clinical microbiology. Washinton DC: American Society for Microbiology, 1981.

Kimura SJ, Thygeson P: The cytology of external ocular disease. Am J Ophthalmol 1955;39:137–145.

Marsh RJ, Fraunfelder FT, McGill JI: Herpetic corneal epithelial disease. Arch Ophthalmol 1976;94:1899–1902.

Naib ZM, Clepper AS, Elliott SR: Exfoliative cytology as an aid in the diagnosis of ophthalmic lesions. Acta Cytol 1967;11:295–303.

Plotkin J, Reynaud A, Okumoto M: Cytologic study of herpetic keratitis: Preparation of corneal scrapings. Arch Ophthalmol 1971;85:597–599.

Spaeth GL: Chronic membranous conjunctivitis. Am J Ophthalmol 1967;64:300–305.

Streeten BW, Streeten EA: "Blue-body" epithelial cell inclusions in conjunctivitis. Ophthalmology 1985;92:575–579.

Thygeson P: Cytology of conjunctival exudates. Am J Ophthalmol 1946;29:1499–1512.

Yoneda C, Dawson CR, Daghfous T, et al.: Cytology as a guide to the presence of chlamydial inclusions in Giemsa-stained conjunctival smears in severe endemic trachoma. Br J Ophthalmol 1975;59:116–124.

5.2 INTERPRETATION OF IMPRESSION CYTOLOGY

To evaluate the process of squamous metaplasia, impression cytology slides are first examined under low power to determine areas with the greatest goblet cell concentration. Using the 40× objective, a differential count is performed to approximate the number of goblet cells per 100 epithelial cells. Morphologic changes in the epithelial cells, such as enlargement, changes in color of cytoplasm, changes in size of nucleus, etc., are noted. The presence or absence of mucus is also noted. A differential count of any inflammatory cells present per 100 epithelial cells is also performed. An interpretation system such as those defined by Tseng or Nelson can be used to evaluate speciemens obtained by impression cytology.

Staging System

The staging system used by Tseng described six different stages in the development of squamous metaplasia based on findings from 35 normal eyes compared with 67 eyes with surface disorders. The system is based on four cytologic features that were correlated with the three major steps in the process of squamous metaplasia. The cytologic features included (1) presence or absence of goblet cells and goblet cell density (GCD). GCD is determined by averaging the numbers of goblet cells counted in ten contiguous microscopic fields at a magnification of 250×, (2) morphologic changes in the nucleus, (3) nucleus/cytoplasm ratios, and (4) metachromatic changes in the color of the cytoplasm and emergence of keratinization. The three major steps in the process of squamous metaplasia were (1) loss of goblet cells, (2) enlargement and flattening of superficial epithelial cells, and (3) keratinization.

The six stages were defined as:

Stage 0—Normal conjunctival epithelium: Moderate numbers of goblet cells scattered among uniform nongoblet epithelial cells that have a blue-green–staining cytoplasm. The nucleus/cytoplasm ratio is approximately 1:1. In interpreting specimens as normal, it is important to note that the normal goblet cell density varies according to the anatomic site of the conjunctiva. For example, the superior bulbar conjunctiva has a lower goblet cell density than the inferior bulbar conjunctiva.

Stage 1—Early loss of goblet cells without keratinization: There is a decrease in the goblet cell density along with a mild enlargement of nongoblet epithelial cells, which have blue-green cytoplasm. The nucleus/cytoplasm ratio ranges from 1:2 to 1:3.

Stage 2—Total loss of goblet cells without keratinization: No goblet cells are seen, and all epithelial cells are moderately enlarged and flattened (squamoid) with the cytoplasm staining a blue-green to mild pinkish color and a nucleus/cytoplasm ratio of 1:4.

Stage 3—Early and mild keratinization: All epithelial cells are markedly squamoid, with a change in the color of the cytoplasm to a pinkish color. Some epithelial cells contained visible keratin filaments. The nucleus/cytoplasm ratio is approximately 1:6 because of flattening of the cytoplasm and mild pyknotic changes in the nucleus.

Stage 4—Moderate keratinization: All epithelial cells are enlarged and squamoid, with pinkish cytoplasm as described above. In addition, more cells contain densely packed keratin filaments, keratohyalin granules, and pyknotic nuclei. The nucleus/cytoplasm ratio is 1:8.

Stage 5—Advanced keratinization: More cells are keratinized with markedly pyknotic nuclei and shrunken cytoplasm with densely packed keratin filaments. In some cells the nucleus may have lysed or is missing.

Grading system

On the basis of a pilot study of 27 eyes with a variety of ocular diagnoses, a grading system was developed by Nelson based on the morphologic appearance of conjunctival epithelial and goblet cells. Impression cytology specimens from bulbar and palpebral conjunctiva were graded on a scale from 0 to 3. Comparison of palpebral and bulbar conjunctival specimens in Nelson's study using this system indicated that the finding of a normal palpebral surface with increased mucus production and goblet cells was consistent with keratoconjunctivitis sicca rather than with a primary ocular surface disease state.

Grade 0: The epithelial cells are small and round with an eosinophilic staining cytoplasm. The nuclei are large and basophilic with a nucleus/cytoplasm ratio of 1:2. There are many goblet cells, which are plump and oval and have an intensely periodic acid-Schiff (PAS)-positive staining cytoplasm.

Grade 1: The epithelial cells are slightly larger, more polygonal in shape, and have an eosinophilic staining cytoplasm. The nuclei are smaller, with a nucleus/cytoplasm ratio of 1:3. The goblet cells are decreased in number; however, they maintain their normal plump, oval shape with intensely PAS-positive staining cytoplasm.

Grade 2: The epithelial cells are larger and polygonal. They are occasionally multinucleated, with a cytoplasm that stains variably. The nuclei are small, with a nucleus/cytoplasm ratio ranging from 1:4 to 1:5. The goblet cells are markedly decreased in number and are smaller, less intensely PAS positive, and have indistinct cell borders.

Grade 3: The epithelial cells are large and polygonal with basophilic staining cytoplasm. The nuclei are small, pyknotic, and completely absent in many cells. The nucleus/cytoplasm ratio is greater than 1:6. Goblet cells are completely absent.

BIBLIOGRAPHY

Blodi BA, Byrne KA, Tabarra KF: Goblet cell populations among patients with inactive trachoma. Int Ophthalmol J 1988;12:41–45.

Nelson JD, Havener VR, Cameron JD: Cellulose acetate impressions of the ocular surface: Dry eye state. Arch Ophthalmol 1983;101:1869–1872.

Tseng SCG: Impression cytology and squamous metaplasia. Ophthalmology 1985; 92:728–733.

Tseng SCG, Maumenee AE, Stark WJ, et al.: Topical retinoid treatment for various dry-eye disorders. Ophthalmology 1985;92:717–733.

Recommendations for Isolation of Microbes from Ocular Specimens

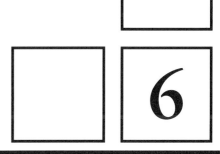

6

Certain media and special culture techniques may be necessary for the isolation of the many bacteria, fungi, and parasites that can be recovered from ocular specimens. Some of these have been discussed in Chapter 3: Setup Procedures and Specimen Collection Protocol. However, because specimens received in the laboratory may be set up by routine microbiologic procedures, the laboratory should have setup requirements easily accessible to assistants and others who may be performing culture inoculation and setups. Some tissues and viral cultures are not directly inoculated bedside and require complete cell culture setup in the laboratory. Parasite culture, if feasible for performance in the reader's laboratory, requires special media and inoculation procedures. Therefore, we have included in this section detailed setup procedures for unusual isolates and Table 6.1 can be placed in a conspicuous position within the setup area as a quick reference of routine culture setup media for ocular cultures.

6.1 RECOMMENDED MEDIA FOR ROUTINE PROCESSING OF OCULAR SPECIMENS

The following table is intended as a guideline for media required for the primary isolation of common isolates in ocular infections. Because some of these sites may be sterile sources and others are nonsterile sources, isolates considered pathogenic differ by site.

Table 6.1
Media and smears to be inoculated for received swabs and aspiration fluids

Source/Site	Routine media	Anaerobe	Fungal	AFB	Smears
Eyelid	BA, CA	If requested	SDA	—	2—Gram, Giemsa
Conjunctiva	BA, CA	If requested	SDA	—	3—Gram, Giemsa, Special
Lacrimal	BA, CA, Thio	ABA	SDA, LJ	LJ	3—Gram, Giemsa, Special
Abscess or drainage	BA, CA, Thio	ABA	SDA	LJ M7H	3—Gram, Giemsa, Special
Cornea	BA, CA, Thio	ABA	SDA	LJ M7H	3-4—Gram, Giemsa, Special
Vitreous, aqueous (anterior chamber)	BA, CA, Thio	*	SDA/LJ	LJ M7H	3-4—Gram, Giemsa, Special
Donor cornea rim and MK media	BA, CA, Thio		SDA		No smears
Donor cornea and MK media	BA, CA, Thio		SDA		No smears

*Anaerobic cultures are automatically performed on intraocular fluids.

Media is abbreviated as follows:

BA = Blood agar
CA = Chocolate blood agar
Thio = Thioglycolate broth culture
SDA = Sabouraud's dextrose agar (Emmons modification)
LJ & M7H = Lowenstein Jensen agar slant & Middlebrook 7H10 or 7H11
TM = Thayer Martin medium or New York City agar
ABA = Anaerobic blood agar (alternatively, Brucella or Laked blood agar may be used)
BHI = Brain heart infusion broth
Gram & Giemsa = Routine smears for ocular cultures
Special = Indicated when one or two extra smears should be made for additional stains that may be required.

Consult Chapter 4 (Staining Procedures for Microscopy) for indication of appropriate special stains. Because these may not be routinely performed in the department, setup personnel should be briefed on fixative requirements for special requests. In general, methanol fixation is recommended for extra smears. Preparation procedures are described in the back of this manual; however, it is recommended to purchase manufacturer-prepared media for quality and consistency.

6.2. PARASITE CULTURE OF FRESHWATER AMOEBAE

Acanthamoeba *and* Naegleria spp
Central nervous system infections caused by free-living amoebae were first recognized in the 1960s. The causative organisms generally fall into the Hartmannella/Acanthamoeba group and are known to cause fatal granulomatous amoebic encephalitis (Garcia 1983). *Naegleria* has been implicated in a fulminant and rapidly fatal meningoencephalitis. Both *Acanthamoeba* and *Naegleria spp* are causative agents in amoebic keratitis. The free-living amoeba may be found in solutions used for soaking and cleaning contact lenses and may survive in water and saline for long periods. Wet mounts from corneal scrapings or anterior chamber fluid can be prepared and stained by calcofluor white followed by a permanent stain to demonstrate cysts or trophozoites (Marines et al. 1987). These are very vision-threatening infections, because antibiotic therapy is often unsuccessful and parasitemia could progress to perforation as a complication of keratitis (Fritsche and Bergeron 1987) and severe life-threatening forms of amoebic encephalitis. Therefore, prompt accurate diagnosis is imperative in these infections of the eye.

Purpose
For the detection and isolation of amoeba using standard nonnutrient culture media with a lawn of *Escherichia coli* and observance of trophozoite activity *in vitro*

Principle
An inoculum obtained from the cornea by tissue biopsy or scraping is applied to an agar containing no nutrients. An amoebic saline is prepared in which live isolates of coliform bacteria are suspended. The mixture is overlayed on agar surface covering the inoculum which provides nutrition for the amoeba. If present, the amoeba will feed on the bacteria and multiply. The plate is observed under slight magnification to detect trophozoite activity by telltale tracks along the surface of the coliform blanket, as shown in Figure 6.1. Once the food supply is exhausted, the amoebae will differentiate into cysts, which then may be stained and undergo electron microscopy to determine the species, based on morphology and ultrastructural details, as shown in Figure 6.2.

Procedure
1. Scrapings or tissue biopsy specimens are obtained according to protocol in Section 3. Microscope slides should be fixed immediately in 95%

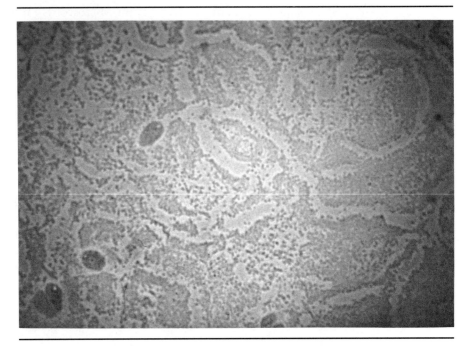

Figure 6.1
Trophozoite tracks on the agar surface as the amoeba feed on the bacteria-seeded nonnutrient agar plate. Dissecting microscope or light microscope using 4× objective at 40× magnification.

ethanol; *Acanthamoeba* cysts left to air dry can become airborne and lost for examination (Baker et al. 1989).

2. A suspension of live *Escherichia coli* (*Enterobacter aerogenes* also has been used) is prepared from colonies less than 18 to 24 hours old using Page's amoebic saline (described in reagent section):
   a. Bring frozen aliquot of Page's saline to room temperature.
   b. Drop 0.5 mL Page's saline into a slant culture of the bacteria. Gently scrape the surface of the culture, allowing it to become suspended in a broth mixture.
   c. Resuspend turbid mixture, using a Pasteur pipet, and withdraw from slant culture.
3. Warm nonnutrient agar plate before inoculating if possible.
4. If contact lens solutions or fluids are cultured, centrifuge specimen at 250g for 10 minutes. With a sterile Pasteur pipet, transfer most of supernatant to a sterile test tube, leaving approximately 1/2 mL sediment that may be inoculated onto a plate to which 3 or 4 drops of bacterial suspension in Page's saline has been precoated.
4. Drop bacterial suspension directly on inoculum of tissue or scraping, allowing it to spread across agar surface entirely (approximately 3 to 4 drops).
5. Seal the plates with 5 or 6 inches of 1-inch ribbon of Parafilm (American National Can, Greenwich, CT) to prevent dehydration.

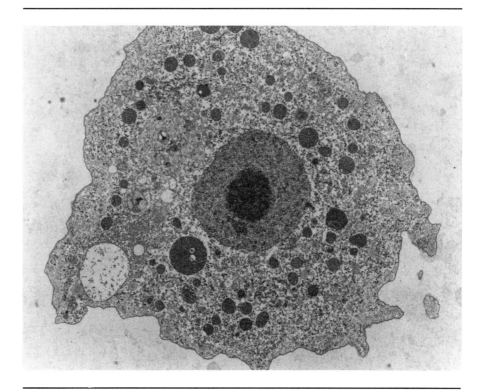

Figure 6.2
Electron microscopy shows ultrastructural details of Acanthamoeba spp *from amoebic keratitis. Courtesy of Romesh K. Gautom, Ph.D., Department of Laboratory Medicine, University of Washington, Seattle, Washington.*

6. Slides may be stained in the Histology Section by Grocott-Methenamine Silver (GMS), calcofluor white, trichrome, or hematoxylin and eosin, depending on the pathologist's or ophthalmologist's preference.

7. Place one plate into a 37°C incubator and the other at 25°C. *Acanthamoeba* grows well at both temperatures, unlike *Naegleria*.

8. Examine plates for amoebae, trophozoites, or cysts, every day for up to 10 days. Telltale tracks can be seen with low magnification of a dissecting microscope or using a 4× objective (40× magnification), as seen in Figure 6.1.

9. On growth of amoebae, a single double-walled cyst may be transferred using a micromanipulator apparatus to a fresh *Escherichia coli*–seeded nonnutrient agar plate for clonal cultures. Subsequent growth on nonnutrient agar plates can then be adapted for axenic growth at 27°C in Trypticase-soy-yeast extract broth (Fritsche et al. 1993).

10. Enflagellation test may be used to differentiate *Naegleria fowleri*, the causative agent in primary amoebic meningoencephalitis. In transformation to a pear-shaped flagellate, two and occasionally three or four flagellae occur during a brief nonfeeding stage before the creature reverts to

a trophozoite. Enflagellation experiments may be conducted as follows (Visvesvara 1992):

  a. If present, amoebae will feed on bacteria until the bacteria are gone, and then the amoebae will differentiate into cysts. Mark the area containing the most trophozoites with a wax pencil.
  b. Using a sterile bacteriologic loop (work under a bacteriologic hood!), transfer several loopfuls of the scraping to a sterile tube containing 2 mL distilled water and incubate at 35° to 37°C, examining periodically.
  c. The presence of flagellates may be seen with an inverted microscope and contractile vacuoles characterizing *N. fowleri* appear as a dark depression inside the trophozoite under 10× or 40× objectives. *Acanthamoeba spp* do not transform to the flagellate state.

11. Electron microscopy is useful in differentiating morphology of ultrastructural details of trophozoites, as seen in Figure 6.2. *Acanthamoeba* are characterized by their double-walled cysts with a wrinkled outer wall (ectocyst) and even round or oval inner wall (endocyst). *Naegleria* trophozoites differentiate into spherical, smooth-walled cysts. Cysts of both are uninucleate.

REFERENCES

Baker AS, Paton B, Haaf J: Ocular infections: Clinical and laboratory considerations. Clin Microbiol Newsl 1989; 11(13):97–101.

Fritsche TR, Bergeron DC: *Acanthamoeba* keratitis. Clin Microbiol Newsl 1987; 9(14).

Fritsche TR, Gautom RK, Seyedirashti S, et al.: Occurrence of bacterial endosymbionts in *Acanthamoeba spp* isolated from corneal and environmental specimens and contact lenses. J Clin Microbiol 1993; 31(5):1122–1126.

Garcia LS: Freshwater amoebae. Clin Microbiol Newsl 1983; 5(16):107–109.

Marines HM, Osato MS, Font RL: The calco-fluor white in the diagnosis of mycotic and acanthamoeba infections of the eye and ocular adnexa. Ophthalmology 1987; 94:23–26.

Visvesvara GS: Parasite culture: *Acanthamoeba* and *Naeglaria*, 7.9.2. In Clinical microbiology procedures handbook, Vol. 2, Washington, D.C.: American Society for Microbiology, 1992.

6.3. MICROSPORIDIA ISOLATION BY CELL CULTURE

Microsporidia are obligate intracellular parasitic protozoa that infect humans and a variety of vertebrate and invertebrate hosts. This emerging pathogen has become an increasingly important cause of keratitis, conjunctivitis, and other opportunistic diseases in patients with human immunodeficiency virus (HIV) and acquired immune deficiency syndrome (AIDS). These include the genuses *Pleistophora, Nosema, Microsporidium,* and *Encephalitozoon* (Schwartz et al. 1993). The source of human infection is unknown, and there is no treatment for either animal or human infections. An antibiotic (fumagillin) has been shown to be effective against nosematosis of honeybees and appears to be parasitostatic against *Encephalitozoon cuniculi in vitro* (Shadduck 1990). These same investigators in 1990 (Shadduck et al. 1990) isolated the microsporidian that they baptized *Nosema corneum* from a human patient by cell culture, according to the following procedure: The patient was treated with topical steroids and broad-spectrum antibiotics, which proved unsuccessful, and he later required a corneal transplant. This case was from an otherwise healthy 45-year-old who was HIV seronegative with no history of ocular trauma and no viral or bacterial pathogens recovered. The microsporidial infection was characterized by a persistent disciform keratitis, recurrent patchy infiltration of the anterior stroma, and iritis. Electron microscopy is necessary to differentiate ultrastructural details of mature spores. Ovoid uninucleate spores measuring 2×1 μm may be present within the cytoplasm of epithelial cells. Polar tubules characteristically coiled and extrusion apparatus may be seen. Additionally, sporonts with diplokarya are significant in *Nosema spp*, helping to differentiate these species.

Specimen
Keratoplasty or corneal biopsies are preferable but scrapings also may be used according to the protocol described in Specimen Collection Techniques. These should be fixed in Hanks' balanced salt solution and transported to the laboratory as soon as possible, up to 12 hours.

Materials
The methods as defined by Shadduck et al. (1990): Two established cell lines may be used with success, SIRC (ATTC 60) derived from rabbit corneal epithelium, and MDCK (ATCC 34) derived from canine kidney both are epithelioid and anchorage dependent.

Eagle's minimum essential medium supplemented with 5% fetal bovine serum and 0.1% gentamicin
0.1% trypsin
0.25% collagenase
25-cm² flasks for cell culture monolayers

Procedure
1. Treat minced pieces of cornea tissue or biopsy specimens with 0.1% trypsin and 0.25% collagenase for 75 minutes at 35° to 37°C.
2. Place on partly confluent cell culture monolayers.
3. Eagle's minimum essential medium supplemented with 5% fetal bovine serum and 0.1% gentamicin is used, and the cultures are incubated at 35° to 37°C in 5% CO_2 in air.
4. After approximately 30 days in culture, SIRC and MDCK cells may have foci of granulated cells, which gradually enlarge over the next 14 days in infected monolayers.
5. Large numbers of small rod-shaped structures may be seen floating in the medium at 60 to 70 days after culture.
6. For electron microscopy, transfer infected monolayers to new dishes, fix for 20 minutes in 2.5% glutaraldehyde in cacodylate buffer (or other suit-

able fixative described in Electron Microscopy), and embed *in situ,* then mark sites.

7. Trim infected sites from the disk of embedded cells and re-embed in capsules for thin sectioning.

Interpretation

Organisms in all stages of development may be seen in the cytoplasm of host cells. Ultrastructurally, the least mature forms (meronts) are characterized by thin, electron-dense outer membranes and poorly developed organelles. Dividing meronts may appear markedly elongated, with a diplokaryon in each future daughter cell in *Nosema corneum.* Polar tubules with up to six or seven coils are characteristic of microsporidia, and mature sporonts have thicker cell walls with a distinct electron-lucent outer zone. Polar tubules of *Nosema connori* and *Microsporidium spp* can have up to ten to eleven coils, differentiating these from *N. corneum* by electron microscopy. Many mature spores may contain only pale amorphous material, having lost their contents. Identical intact and degenerative spores may be seen in original biopsy tissue and are useful in confirming culture-true-positives.

REFERENCES

Schwartz DA, Visvesvara GS, Diesenhouse MC, et al.: Pathologic features and immunofluorescent antibody demonstration of ocular microsporidiosis in seven patients with AIDS. AM J Ophthalmol 1993; 115(3):285–292.

Shadduck JA: Effect of fumagillin on in vitro multiplication of *Encephalitozoon cuniculi.* J Protozool 1980; 27:202–208.

Shadduck JA, Meccoli RA, Davis R, Font RL: Isolation of a microsporidian from a human patient. J Infect Dis 1990; 162:773–776.

6.4. CHLAMYDIA CULTURE IN CYCLOHEXIMIDE-TREATED McCOY CELLS

McCoy cells supplemented with fetal bovine serum (FBS) are optimally acceptable for the isolation and identification of *Chlamydia trachomatis* from ocular specimens. Potential alternate sera and synthetic serum substitutes have been examined; however, comparative assay results of growth rates did not equal that of FBS (Truant and Hepler 1983), the rationale being that the early developmental stage of the bovine fetuses immune system dictated minimal immune responsiveness. In addition, the restricted exposure time of the donor animal to exogenous microorganisms present *in utero* further implied low-level circulating antibodies. FBS may be superior to alternate seras for the isolation of a number of serotypes of *C. trachomatis.*

Preparation of Cell Monolayers

1. McCoy cells are propagated as monolayers in 25-cm² tissue culture flasks. Growth medium: Eagle's minimal essential medium (MEM), supplemented

with 10% fetal calf serum, 1% glutamine, 1% gentamicin (10 μg/mL). Adjust pH to 7.4 with 7.5% sodium bicarbonate.

2. Cells are passaged 1:4 by routine trypsinization.
3. Incubate newly passaged cultures for 4 days at 37°C to form a monolayer.
4. Remove growth medium and wash cells in phosphate-buffered saline.
5. Add 2-mL 0.25% trypsin; swirl over the monolayer so that all cells have been exposed, then remove the trypsin. Incubate the flask at 35° to 37°C for 3 to 5 minutes or until the cell sheet begins to fall in the flask.
6. Resuspend, count, and dilute the cells in growth medium to a concentration of 2×10^5 cells/mL.
7. Transfer 1.0 mL diluted cells into three shell vials containing a coverslip.
8. Incubate shell vials for 24 hours to form confluent monolayers.
9. Remove the growth medium from the vials. The McCoy cells are then ready for inoculation.

Commonly used cell lines

McCoy cells are the most widely used but are not notably superior to other cell lines. McCoy cells are believed to have originated from human synovial cells, but the McCoy cells now used in laboratories are mouse fibroblasts.

HeLa 229 cells originated from human cervical cancer.

BHK 21 cells were derived from baby hamster kidney.

L929 cells derived from mouse connective tissue.

BGMK cells derived from African green monkey kidney.

Inoculation procedure

1. Mix gently the specimen collected in Chlamydial Transport Medium (CTM), then transfer 1.0 mL specimen from CTM into three tubes containing coverslips.
2. Centrifuge the tubes at 3000g for 1 hour at room temperature to obtain a maximum interaction between infectious *Chlamydia* and host cell.
3. After centrifugation, incubate the three tubes at 37°C for 1 hour to prolong the attachment–phagocytosis phase.
4. After incubation, discard the CTM and add 1.0 mL isolation medium (MEM, 2% FBS, 3 μm/mL glucose, 10 μg/mL gentamicin) supplemented with 0.1 mL (20 mg/L) of cycloheximide to each of the three tubes to inhibit the growth of McCoy cells while the glucose promotes growth of *Chlamydia trachomatis*.
5. The cultures are then incubated at 37°C in 5% CO_2 for 3 days.
6. After incubation, one of the three tubes is subjected to staining for detection of intracytoplasmic inclusions of *Chlamydia trachomatis* by Microtrak (Syra Co., San Jose, CA) fluorescein-labeled monoclonal antibody method described in Section 4.2.6.
7. The two remaining tubes are reincubated for an additional 24 hours, then the second tube is subjected to staining.
8. The third tube is used for passage to form another two cultures (handled as already described).

Limitations

In some cases, direct fluorescence antibody tests (DFA) may yield positive results when the culture is negative. However, these have not been evaluated for children, complicated by evidence that asymptomatic infections can be acquired perinatally and may persist for several months in the absence of symptoms or specific therapy (Porder et al. 1989). Exclusive testing by enzymatic methods such as Chlamydiazyme (Abbott, Chicago, IL) enzyme immunoassay (EIA) should never take the place of culture or DFA because of low sensitivity and specificity.

REFERENCES

Porder K.: Lack of specificity of Chlamydiazyme for detection of vaginal chlamydial infection in prepubertal girls. Pediatr Infect Dis J 1989; 8:358–360.
Truant AL, Hepler RE: Serum supplements for the propagation of HeLa-229 and McCoy cells. Clin Microbiol Newsl 1983; 5(2):9–11.

BIBLIOGRAPHY

Lennette EH: Laboratory diagnosis of viral infections. New York: Marcel Dekker, 1985:199–203.
LaScolea LJ: Chlamydial infections: The mother-infant connection. Clin Microbiol Newsletter, 1986, 8:77.
Oriel J, Ridgway GL: Genital infection by *Chlamydia trachomatis*. London: Edward Arnold, 1982:114–115.
Sommerville RG: Essential clinical virology. London: Blackwell Scientific Publications, 1986:14–19.

6.5. HERPES SIMPLEX VIRUS (HSV1 AND HSV2) CELL CULTURE

Herpes simplex virus (HSV) can be divided into type 1 and type 2 based on antigenic, biochemical, and biologic differences. A rapid diagnostic method is essential for adequate evaluation of patients with suspected herpetic keratitis and conjunctivitis. Use of fluorescein-labeled monoclonal antibodies in a shell vial assay provides rapid detection of HSV. Serious, life-threatening illnesses caused by HSV occur, and neonatal HSV infections occur when newborns contract HSV during vaginal delivery. Approximately 85% of babies who acquire disseminated neonatal HSV infection die of their disease, and neurologic sequelae are frequent in survivors (Mayo 1983). Herpesvirus B (HVB), also known as *Herpesvirus simiae*, though rare (fewer than 30 human cases), is almost always fatal, and individuals working directly with carrier monkeys or their tissues have increased risk (Snook 1992). Three different drugs, acyclovir, vidarabine, and foscarnet, are available to treat HSV infections (Abramowicz 1990). However, a series of case reports, beginning in 1987, has indicated that in immunocompromised patients, resistant HSV can be associated with severe, progressive mucocutaneous infection and conjunctivitis that does not respond to acyclovir, which is commonly used to treat these infections (Erlich et al.

1989). There is some speculation whether the HSV-resistant variants remain virulent, because resistance is caused by changes in essential viral enzymes. Although not yet determined, this may necessitate susceptibility testing in the future. Herpesvirus cell culture and differentiation of HSV1 and HSV2 are helpful in establishing the definitive diagnosis in ocular infections.

Cell lines

MRC-5 cell cultures are very susceptible to infection by HSV and produce consistent characteristic cytopathic effect. Monolayers of MRC-5 cells are grown on coverslips in shell vials. Ocular clinical specimens are inoculated directly into the vials and incubated for a minimum of 16 hours before being stained with fluorescein-labeled monoclonal antibodies used for detection and differentiation of HSV1 and HSV2.

Other commonly used cell lines

1. **Vero cells:** derived from African green monkey kidney cells
2. **HeLa cells:** derived from human carcinoma of the cervix
3. **HEp-2 cells:** derived from larynx

Treatment of cells

1. One milliliter MRC-5 cells (concentration 50,000 cells/mL) suspended in growth medium: Eagle's MEM, supplemented with 10% fetal calf serum, 1% glutamine, 1% gentamicin (10 µg/mL), adjust pH to 7.4 with 7.5% sodium bicarbonate.
2. Seed onto coverslips in one dram shell vials and incubate at 35° to 37°C for 24 hours to form monolayers. Note: Preseeded vials may be purchased commercially from Baxter (Bartels Diagnostics Inc., Issaquah, WA).
3. Aspirate the medium from shell vials and inoculate 0.2 mL specimen into each vial.
4. Cap vials and centrifuge at 700g for 40 minutes at room temperature.
5. After centrifugation, add 1 mL culture medium and incubate at 35° to 37°C.
6. Incubate culture for at least 16 hours, then aspirate most of the medium from each vial into a flask containing bleach. Do not allow monolayers to dry.
7. After removal of growth medium, wash coverslips twice in phosphate-buffered saline (PBS).
8. Aspirate PBS from the second wash and fix the cells to the coverslip using cold acetone, filling the vial completely. Leave for 20 minutes, then aspirate the acetone into a flask of bleach. Evaporate the acetone under a fume hood.
9. Add 200 µL HSV 1 monoclonal antibody to one shell vial and repeat for HSV2 monoclonal antibody to the other paired shell vial, ensuring complete coverage.
10. Cover the vials to prevent evaporation, then incubate at 35° to 37°C for 30 minutes.
11. Wash the coverslips 2 times in PBS to wash away any unbound antibody.
12. Mount the coverslips cell side down on a slide using fluorescent antibody mounting fluid.

13. Read at 400×, scanning entire coverslip for characteristic fluorescence staining of at least one cell, according to stain procedure described in Chapter 4.

Interpretation

Apple-green fluorescence ranges from a fine granular to a coarse stippled appearance. As in the standard procedure for HSV fluorescence method, use the positive control as a reference for expected stain reactions and a negative control to check reagent and technique. Optimal performance of this test is dependent on proper inoculation technique, collection, and transport of an adequate patient specimen.

Vero cell culture (alternative method for longer incubation)

1. Transfer 1.0 mL, 3- to 4-day-old cell cultures of Vero splitted cells into two tubes.
2. Incubate tubes for 24 hours at 37°C to have a confluent monolayer.
3. Discard the growth medium from the tubes. The Vero cells are then ready for inoculation.

Inoculation procedure

1. Into two tubes containing confluent monolayer of Vero cells, inoculate 0.1 mL clinical specimen from viral transport medium into one tube for test; the other tube may serve as an uninoculated control.
2. Virus is allowed to absorb by incubating the cultures at 37°C for 1 hour.
3. Maintenance medium 1.0 mL is added to the culture tubes, which are then incubated at 37°C.
4. Examine microscopically and observe daily for cytopathic effect (CPE) for up to 7 days.

NOTE: The duration before CPE is observed depends on the virus titer in the clinical specimen. High titers of HSV show extensive CPE often demonstrable in a matter of 24 hours. Most isolates produce CPE by 3 to 4 days; however, cultures should be observed for 6 to 7 days.

Interpretation

Herpes simplex virus produces a specific pattern of CPE with large, round, balloon cells or sometimes as formations of multinucleated syncytial giant cells. If no CPE is observed by 7 days, the cultures can be frozen and thawed 3 times in an alcohol–dry ice bath, and 0.1 mL lysate can be used to inoculate fresh cell monolayers. These cultures are observed for an additional 7 days and may be used for the passage procedure in viral culture.

REFERENCES

Abramowicz M: Drugs for viral infections. Med Lett 1990; 32:73–78.

Erlich KS, Mills J, Chati FP et al.: Acyclovir resistant herpes simplex virus infections in patients with the acquired immunodeficiency syndrome. N Engl J Med 1989; 320:293–296.

Mayo DR: Laboratory diagnosis of herpes simplex. Clin Microbiol Newsl 1983; 5(4):21–23.

Snook SS: Herpesvirus B. Clin Microbiol Newsl 1992; 14(6):41–43.

BIBLIOGRAPHY

Costello MJ, Morrow SL, Laney S, et al. Guidelines for specimen collection, transportation, and test selection. Lab Med. 1993; 24:19.

Gomerville RG: Essential clinical virology. London: Blackwell Scientific Publications, 1986:14–19.

Henry JB: Clinical diagnosis and management by laboratory methods. Volume 2. 16th Edition. Philadelphia: W.B. Saunders, 1979:1838.

Lenette EH: Laboratory diagnosis of viral infections. New York: Marcel Dekker, 1985:318–319.

6.6 ADENOVIRUS CELL CULTURE

Adenovirus is a double-stranded DNA virus. Currently, forty-two serotypes of human origin have been classified by serology and DNA electrophoretyping, and several additions are being considered. They are common human pathogens and cause clinical infections of the eye, respiratory, gastrointestinal, and urinary tract. Conjunctivitis is the primary ocular syndrome caused by adenovirus infection. Adenoviruses are thought to be responsible for approximately 20% of conjunctivitis cases and may be seen in one of two forms:

Pharyngoconjunctival fever is a respiratory illness with symptoms of fever/chills, pharyngitis, nonproductive cough, myalgia, etc., seen primarily in school-aged children, although sporadic cases have been reported in other age groups. In two-thirds of cases, there is an associated conjunctivitis that is usually unilateral. It is highly contagious and is spread primarily by droplet transmission. Outbreaks during summer months as a result of spread in swimming pools are common. The incubation period for pharyngoconjunctival fever is approximately 5 to 6 days, and virus shedding may occur for up to 10 days. Pharyngoconjunctival fever is primarily caused by serotypes 3, 7, and 14, although serotypes 1, 2, 4, and 6 have also been observed.

Epidemic keratoconjunctivitis (EKC) is an acute follicular conjunctivitis with preauricular adenopathy and occasionally with true or pseudomembrane formation. The eye infection also can be accompanied by respiratory illness. The infection is highly contagious and can affect individuals of any age. Hand–eye contact is the most common mode of transmission. Contaminated eye instruments and eye solutions as well as towels are also sources of infection. The disease process is self-limited, with resolution in approximately 2 weeks. Complications can include a superficial punctate keratitis followed by subepithelial opacities that can persist for many months and can interfere with vision. The principle adenovirus serotypes involved are 8, 11, 19, and 37, although others have been reported. The diagnosis is usually based solely on clinical presentation, although laboratory studies may be helpful in cases where the diagnosis is in question.

Clinical specimens can be examined directly by electron microscopy, indirect fluorescent antibody procedures, *in situ* hybridization, enzyme immunoassay, etc. However, cell culture isolation is considered to be a sensitive technique and is currently the method of choice for use in most clinical laboratories. A procedure for cell culture isolation follows.

Cells

Most human adenoviruses of serotypes 1 through 39 replicate and produce cytopathic effects best in A549 (human embryonic kidney) cells. Some strains also grow well in human cell lines (HeLa, HEp-2, MRC-5) and primary monkey kidney (PMK) cells. The enteric enteroviruses, serotypes 40 and 41, do not grow well in cell culture. Human embryonic kidney cells that have been transformed with type 5 adenovirus (239 cells) are most sensitive for the isolation of these serotypes.

Specimen

Conjunctival specimens can be taken using a sterile Kimura spatula or a swab premoistened with saline. The lower cul-de-sac is the usual sampling site and is where follicles are best appreciated. In cases of corneal involvement, corneal scrapings also can be taken with a Kimura spatula. The swab or conjunctival or corneal cells obtained by scraping are placed in viral transport medium. As with other infectious agents, isolation rates are increased by proper specimen collection and handling. Ideal specimens are obtained early in the disease course and are transported to the clinical laboratory promptly. Specimens that cannot be transported immediately should be held at 4°C.

Inoculation procedure

1. Specimens are preferably inoculated onto susceptible cells on the same day that they are received.
2. Swabs in transport medium (2.5 mL) are vortexed and material from the swab is expressed into the medium.
3. Inoculate 200 μL specimen into each tube of A549 cells.
4. Incubate at 35°C for 1 hour to allow the virus to adsorb, then add 1 mL culture medium to each tube. Incubate the A549 tubes in slanting racks at 35°C.
5. To minimize any toxic effects of the specimen, the medium should be changed within 48 hours after inoculation. Subsequently, the medium should be changed every 2 to 3 days for cultures of continuous cell lines or every 7 to 10 days for primary and diploid cell cultures.
6. Examine the cultures microscopically for the presence of cytopathic effect at 24 hours and 2 to 3 times/week for at least 14 days (some laboratories prefer to hold adenovirus cultures for 28 days).

Interpretation

The time of appearance of cytopathic effect depends on the serotype of adenovirus and on the amount of virus present in the specimen. Typical cytopathic effect appears on average at about 6 days after inoculation. Members of the subgenus D may take up to 28 days to show cytopathic effect or may only appear after subpassage.

Characteristic cytopathic effect is seen as swollen infected cells in grapelike clusters. Especially with A549 cells, cytoplasmic stranding may occur, giving a lattice appearance to the monolayer.

Identification of the isolate

Cultures that are presumptive for adenovirus by the presence of characteristic cytopathic effect must be confirmed by additional tests. Immunofluorescence techniques (IF) (Bion Enterprises, Park Ridge, IL), enzyme-linked immunosorbent assay (ELISA) (Vidas Assay, BioMerieux, Hazelwood, MO), complement fixation, and several other techniques are available for confirmation testing. Cell cultures that show 25% to 50% cytopathic effect can be identified by IF or ELISA. Other identification techniques work best if 75% to 100% of the monolayer is affected. For most clinical purposes, confirmation of the isolate as belonging to the genus adenovirus without serotype differentiation is sufficient. If necessary, the serotype can be determined by neutralization tests.

BIBLIOGRAPHY

Baron EJ, Peterson LR, Finegold SM (eds.): Bailey and Scott's diagnostic microbiology, 9th Edition. Chapter 43: Laboratory Methods in Basic Virology. St. Louis: C.V. Mosby, 1994, p. 634–688.

Lennette EH: Laboratory diagnosis of viral infections, 2nd edition. New York: Marcel Dekker, 1991.

Incubation and Processing of Cultures in the Laboratory

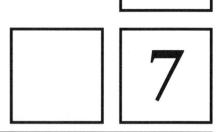

Once the specimen has been set up by the ophthalmologist, and received in the microbiology laboratory, the plates and tubes or broths must be placed in the appropriate atmosphere and temperature for isolation. Occasionally it is necessary to process specimens that were not set up bedside and come to the microbiology laboratory on swabs or in syringes.

Once growth is achieved, the careful workup and processing of the isolates begins. Because ocular pathogens differ somewhat from wound and other body sites encountered in routine microbiology, it is imperative that quantities and sometimes nonpathogenic organisms from these cultures not be dismissed. For instance, there is no "light, moderate, or other normal flora" from a cornea or intraocular fluid.

It is important that the microbiologist become familiar with the significance of certain isolates and be aware of disease processes in which an organism considered "normal flora" is causing an infection in the eye. A glossary of terms and diagnoses are provided and should be consulted. Good communication with the ophthalmologist is helpful in the workup and subsequent antibiotic sensitivity tests when in doubt.

7.1 INCUBATION REQUIREMENTS

7.1.1 Conditions

1. Temperature
1. Aerobic and facultatively anaerobic bacteria: 35°C (5% to 10% CO_2)

94

2. Anaerobic bacteria and *Actinomyces spp:* 35°C (anaerobic system)
3. *Mycobacteria* and *Nocardia spp:* 35°C (5% to 10% CO_2)
4. *Acanthamoeba* and *Naeglaria spp:* 35°C and 27°C
5. *Neisseriae, Branhamella spp:* 35°C (5% to 10% CO_2)
6. Fungi: 25° to 30°C
7. Viruses and Microsporidia: 35° to 37°C (5% to 10% CO_2)
8. *Chlamydia trachomatis:* 35° to 37°C (5% to 10% CO_2)

2. Atmosphere
1. Cultured plates, that is, blood agar, chocolate agar, and Lowenstein-Jensen are incubated in a CO_2 incubator.
2. Broth media, that is, cooked meat broth, thioglycolate broth, are incubated in a regular non-CO_2 incubator.
3. Sabouraud's dextrose agar for fungus is incubated in a regular non-CO_2 incubator.
4. Anaerobic blood agar is incubated anaerobically in a jar containing catalyst, disposable indicator, and disposable $H_2 + CO_2$ generator envelope.

3. Length of Incubation
1. Bacterial cultures
   Sterile sources .... 7 days
   Nonsterile sources.. 3 days
2. Anaerobic cultures .... 14 days
3. Fungal cultures .... 21 days
4. Mycobacterium cultures .... 8 weeks
5. *Acanthamoeba* and *Naegleria* cultures................................. 7 to 10 days
6. Gonococcus cultures .... 5 days
7. Viral cultures .... 14 days
8. *Chlamydia* cultures.. 3 to 4 days
9. Microsporidia cultures.. 30 to 60 days

7.2 PROCESSING OF SPECIMEN

7.2.1. Receiving of Specimen

1. Match labeled specimen with completed Microbiology form.
2. The patient name and number must match on both specimen and requisition form.
3. Check the requisition form to see that the information is according to Chapter 2 of this manual. If not complete, return or call to sender for completion. Hold specimen under appropriate conditions.
4. Label all plates, tubes, and slides with accession number.
5. Include patient number and date on all plates, tubes, and slides.

7.2.2. Culturing of Specimen

1. Received on swabs

Inoculated media is listed for type of culture requested (i.e., routine, anaerobic, fungal, acid-fast bacillus (AFB): refer to Recommended Media for Ocular Specimens. Separate swabs must be submitted with a separate requisition form for each type of culture and smear.

2. Received plates, broth

Blood agar, chocolate agar, and thioglycolate broth: incubate at 35°C in CO_2 incubator.

Anaerobic blood agar: incubate in anaerobic GasPak jar at 35°C in a non-CO_2 incubator.

Sabouraud's agar plate: incubate at room temperature or preferably in a 27° to 30°C incubator.

Lowenstein-Jensen medium: incubate at 35°C in CO_2 incubator.

Acanthamoeba/Naegleria culture plates: incubate one plate at 35° to 37°C and the other at 27° to 30°C non-CO_2 incubators.

3. Received aspiration fluids

All fluids should be set up and inoculated directly onto culture media by the attending ophthalmologist if possible. Plates and broth for anaerobic isolation should be incubated within 1 hour of collection.

Fluids received in **stoppered** syringe transported to the laboratory should be set up **immediately** as follows:

1. Approximate volume received: make sure there is enough volume, 2 to 3 drops maximum for each of the following media and slides. If there is very little material, do not inoculate all those mentioned in the following; proceed to step 5 below.
2. Expel a few drops to each of the plated media, making sure there is enough fluid for broths and smears. Drops should fall freely (do not touch media) directly to center of dish. Inoculate blood agar (2), chocolate agar (1), Sabouraud's agar (1).
2. Inject a few to several drops into thioglycolate (2 tubes), and cooked meat broth (1).
3. Prepare three to four smears from remaining fluid, allow to air dry.
4. Inoculate blood agar (1) immediately in an anaerobe jar, keeping plate upright so as not to leak fluid into lid, place in 35°C.
5. If volume is not sufficient for inoculation to all of the above, then the following will provide the most critical information: chocolate agar (1), thioglycolate (1), Sabouraud's agar (1), smear (1).

4. Received tissues or biopsy materials

Materials received for microbiologic investigation will be ground before inoculation, using a sterile tissue grinder with a few drops tryptic soy broth added (up to 1 mL), pulverized or liquefied as much as possible.

Culture media is setup the same as fluids (steps 1 to 5), using a sterile Pasteur pipet in place of needle and syringe.

5. Received Donor Corneal Rims/Media
Samples of bathing medium should be inoculated to either supplemented thioglycolate medium or brain heart infusion broth enriched with 0.5% beef extract in dilutions of 1:10 and 1:100 to eliminate the activity of the antibiotics. The unused corneoscleral tissue can be emulsified and inoculated as for other tissues.

7.3 READING/PROCESSING OF CULTURES

Routine cultures
All plates are to be examined daily for growth, preferably with magnification. Broth cultures are to be observed daily with a blind-sub to an anaerobic blood agar and aerobic blood agar/chocolate agar done at 24 hours.

Positive growth is to be quantitated and identified with sensitivities performed on significant isolates. Turbidity in broth culture is to be Gram stained for preliminary identification and subcultured aerobically for isolation and identification (and susceptibility testing when appropriate).

Plates showing no growth under daily observation are to be held for 3 days before discarding as "No Growth." Broths are to be held 5 days before discarding as "No Growth."

Written preliminary reports should go out at 24 hours whether positive or negative. Interim written reports should go out on all negative cultures turned positive if significance warrants workup, thus delaying the final report. All significant positive cultures (i.e., corneal, intraocular fluids, positive cultures) must be called immediately to the physician.

Fungal cultures
Fungal plates/tubes (Sabouraud's/Lowenstein-Jensen) are to be observed daily for the first week, because *Aspergillus spp* may be positive within 24 to 48 hours, as shown in Plate 46, as may *Fusarium spp,* the two most common causes of mycotic keratitis. Significant growth (i.e., all fungi growing in the inoculated area of the agar or true pathogen) should be called immediately to the physician with a written preliminary "Final report to follow."

Cultures showing no growth should be followed by a written report at 7 days and final report "No Growth" at 3 weeks. Lactophenol cotton blue wet preparations are recommended for initial observation of fungi for spores. *Fusarium spp* are white, cottony-woolly, sometimes becoming pink or purple in the substrate. Microscopically the mycelia are septate and phialides are borne singly or in packed groups (sporodochia). Macroconidia are sickled or recognizable by their banana shape, with pointed ends as shown in Figure 7.1. *Aspergillus spp* (*A. flavus, A. fumigatus, A. niger, A. terreus*) are more common in Saudia Arabia, India, and the agricultural regions of the United States (Khairallah et al. 1992) and are recognized by their conidial apparatus with terminal swelling of the conidiophore bearing fruitful chains of conidia and secondary sterig-

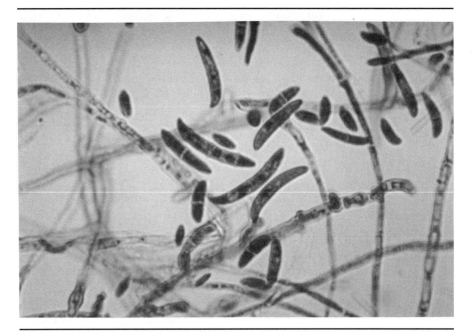

Figure 7.1
Lactophenol-cotton-blue (LCB)–stained wet preparation of plate growth from Fusarium solani *keratitis has septated macroconidia, sickle shape, with pointed ends. 400×
magnification.*

mata, as can be seen in Figure 7.2 of a mature and young development of primary sterigmata. It is important to view some fungi immediately before the hyphae become old and the spores or conidia have fallen free to differentiate species. Reference laboratories should be used whenever unusual isolates are encountered, or regularly, depending on the mycologic expertise of the microbiology staff.

Anaerobic cultures
Blood agar plates are to be read after 48 hours in the anaerobic GasPak jar. Negative plates must be reincubated for an additional 12 days and checked every 72 hours for visible growth before discarding as "No Growth." Positive isolates must be Gram stained and subcultured anaerobically and aerobically. Significant positives (i.e., anaerobic blood agar [ABA] positive with routine culture negative, ABA positive with typical morphology of true anaerobe) are to be identified with sensitivities and called immediately with a written report.

Broths that are incubated under anaerobic conditions are to be observed for turbidity every 72 hours. Subculture onto two blood agar plates if broth shows visible signs of turbidity and reincubate anaerobically (1 BA) and aerobically (1 BA). The second blood agar plate is used to rule out facultative growth of aerobes, and the first is processed in the same manner as described (Perry et al. 1982).

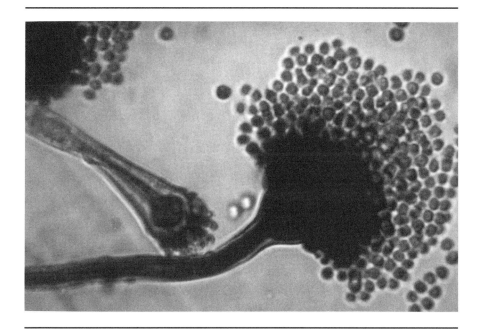

Figure 7.2
LCB-stained wet preparation from Aspergillus flavus *exhibit young primary and mature secondary sterigmata bearing fruitful chains of conidia. 1,000× magnification.*

Acid-fast bacillus (AFB) cultures

Lowenstein-Jensen and Middlebrook agars must be observed weekly for growth. *Mycobacterium tuberculosis* may appear within the first few weeks and grows well on Lowenstein-Jensen media, as shown in Plate 47. All growth is to be Gram stained and acid-fast or Auramine-Rhodamine stained. Identify AFB-positive or positive fluorescence isolates and all Actinomycetes that may also be present on anaereobically incubated blood agars, as shown in Plate 48, pitting the agar.

All significant positive cultures (i.e., AFB or Actinomycetes) should be called, followed by a written report. Negative cultures should have a preliminary interim "No Growth" report sent at 2 weeks. Final No Growth reports are sent at 8 weeks.

Acanthamoeba and Naegleria cultures

To detect *Acanthamoeba* and *Naegleria,* agar plates should be incubated at 35° to 37°C and 27° to 30°C and examined daily with a dissecting (stereoscope) microscope by oblique (450) illumination or low-power objective of 4× or 2× to visualize the fine serpentine indentation lines on the surface of the media, as seen in Figure 6.1. Agar material of positive cultures should be removed with a thin-walled capillary pipet or fine spatula and transferred to nonnutrient agar with an overlay of young *Escherichia coli.*

Another specimen should be taken from culture plate and placed onto two clean glass slides. Slides may be stained by hematoxylin and eosin or calcofluor stains and examined for the presence of cysts and trophozoites resembling *Acanthamoeba* or *Naegleria spp.*

Gonococcus/meningococcus cultures

Thayer Martin agar is to be observed daily for growth. All growth is to be Gram stained and tested by sugar utilization identification schemes, followed by serotyping. Report all positives as soon as possible. "No Growth" reports are sent after 5 days.

7.4 INTERPRETATION OF CULTURE GROWTH BY SPECIMEN

Lid and conjunctiva

Interpretation of growth of various organisms requires familiarity with the normal indigenous microflora. The following are the normal conjunctival flora:

1. *Staphylococcus epidermidis* .... 75% to 90%
2. *Corynebacterium spp* .... 20% to 75%
3. *Propionibacterium acnes* 50%
4. *Staphylococcus aureus* .... 25% to 40%
5. *Streptococcus sp* .... 2% to 10%
6. *Branhamella catarrhalis* 5%
7. Gram-negative rods .... 0% to 5%

Selection of colonies for the identification and antibiotic susceptibility testing is based on the clinical diagnosis, and in unilateral infections, the type of growth from the contralateral eye.

Quantitation of colony growth on lid and conjunctiva

Findings	Grade
Less than 15 colonies	Scant Growth
More than 15 colonies isolated in primary streak area	Light growth
More than 50 colonies in primary secondary and in the third streak	Moderate growth
Mass coalescence in entire area (more than 150 colonies)	Heavy growth

Cornea

Growth outside the inoculation marks (C streaks) on solid medium should be disregarded as contamination and circled with a wax pencil on the reverse of the plate. Indigenous organisms in the preocular tear film can be cultured in infectious and noninfectious keratitis and will appear on the inoculation marks on solid media. Recognition of the indigenous flora is aided by sparse growth and the appearance of the same organisms in the culture of the conjunctiva. The number of colonies are counted, and the number per C streak and the number of streaks yielding growth are recorded. For the anaerobic culture, if limited to inoculated supplemented thioglycolate broth, aerobic and anaerobic subcultures must be made when broth exhibits turbidity or evidence of bacterial growth. Most fungi causing keratitis can be detected within 5 to 7 days; however, ocular cultures should be kept for a minimum of 3 weeks.

Quantitation of colony growth of corneal cultures findings
Few colonies (fewer than 10) .... scant growth
Growth on half of inoculum .... light growth
Growth on half of inoculum but all streaks......................... moderate growth
Growth on all inoculums .... heavy growth

Identify with sensitivities all bacterial isolates. Identify all fungal, Actinomycetes, or AFB isolates.

Intraocular fluids
Cultures from direct inoculation of small volumes of aqueous (0.1 to 0.2 mL) or vitreous (0.5 to 2.0 mL) fluid are handled in the same manner as corneal cultures. Plate contaminants can be recognized as colony growth away from the fluid impression zones. Quantitation of colony growth is the same as cornea. All isolates from anterior chamber or vitreous should be identified with sensitivities.

Lacrimal discharge/abscess drainage
Pure growth of a true pathogen (at any quantity) is to be identified with sensitivities. Moderate growth of two potentially pathogenic organisms are to be identified with sensitivities. In moderate to heavy growth of more than three organisms, identify organisms, perform sensitivities, and then report identity as a mixed culture. Growth of any quantity of microorganism if the initial Gram-stained clinical specimens showed microorganisms intracellularly are to be identified with sensitivities.

Donor corneal rim/media/tissue/foreign bodies
All positive growth is to be identified with sensitivities and called immediately to the physician, followed by a written report. This is imperative because this is a postoperative workup for material that has already been used for transplant.

REFERENCES

Khairallah S, Byrne K, Tabbara KF: Fungal keratitis in Saudi Arabia. Doc Ophthalmol 1992;79:269–276.

Perry LD, Brinser JH, Kolodner H: Anaerobic corneal ulcers. Ophthalmology 1982;89(6):636–641.

BIBLIOGRAPHY

Baker AS, Paton BP, Haaf J: Ocular infections: Clinical laboratory considerations. Clin Microbiol Newsl 1989;11(13):97–101.

Henry JB (ed.): Clinical diagnosis and management by laboratory methods. 18th Edition. Philadelphia: W.B. Saunders, 1991.

Kent, PT, Kubica GP: Public health mycobacteriology: A guide for the level III laboratory. Atlanta, GA: U.S. Department of Health and Human Services, Centers for Disease Control, 1985.

Koneman EW, Allen S, Dowell VR, Sommers HM: Color atlas of clinical microbiology. 4th Edition. Philadelphia: J.B. Lippincott, 1992.

Mandell GL, Douglas RG Jr, Bennett JE (eds.): Principles and practice of infectious diseases. 3rd Edition. New York: Churchill Livingstone, 1990.

Tabbara KF, Hyndiuk RA: Infections of the eye. Boston: Little, Brown, 1986.

7.5 QUANTITATIVE OCULAR MICROBIOLOGY

The ocular microbiology procedures routinely used in clinical laboratories permit only semiquantitative evaluation of ocular cultures. The indication of light, moderate, or heavy growth is sufficient to indicate clinical significance or insignificance of a particular isolate. In research studies, however, particularly those designed to evaluate new antibacterial agents or new therapeutic regimens, it becomes necessary to employ accurate methods that quantitate numbers of colony growth or "colony-forming units" (CFUs). A quantitative method that has gained widespread acceptance for use in clinical studies has been described by Cagle and Abshire (1981). This method works for specimens taken from the eyelids or conjunctivae. It is critical that cultures be taken in exactly the same manner each time for result comparison studies.

Conjunctival cultures
1. Moisten calcium alginate swab in sterile liquid broth.
2. Starting in the lower conjunctival fornix at the nasal margin, pass swab along the conjunctiva to the temporal margin and back again while rotating the swab 180 degrees.
3. Immediately place swab in a tube of 0.3 mL transport buffer (BSS, Alcon Labs, Fort Worth, Texas) and five glass beads.
4. Specimens may be held at 4°C for up to 4 hours.

Eyelid Cultures
Processed in the same manner as conjunctiva but rather running a moistened calcium alginate swab **along the eyelash margin** from the nasal edge to the temporal edge and back again.

Processing specimens
1. Gently vortex the transport tube for 1 to 2 minutes with addition of 1.5 mL loosening fluid (Eagle-Earle Minimum Essential Medium without L-glutamine).

2. Let stand at room temperature for 15 minutes.
3. Vortex vigorously for 1 minute to loosen strands of swab material.
4. Add 1.3 mL dissolving fluid (2.5% sodium metaphosphate, pH 7.0 to 7.2).
5. Vortex tube again vigorously for 1 minute to dissolve the calcium strands.
6. Prepare 1-mL aliquots for inoculation onto the following media (spreading evenly with sterile bent glass rod):
   a. Blood agar (1)
   b. Chocolate agar (1)

   Note: Some investigators (Folkens et al. In press) expand the plating procedure to include four serial tenfold dilutions of the specimen.
   A. A 10^1 dilution is simulated by plating 0.1 mL undiluted specimen.
   B. Remaining dilutions are prepared in normal saline and 1-mL aliquot dilutions are plated onto blood and chocolate agar plates.
7. Incubate all plates at 35° to 37°C.
8. The numbers of colony growth are counted and the plating dilution factor is applied according to the dilution factor (i.e., multiply by 10 if 0.1 mL was plated, and 10 for the first plate of a 10^1 dilution, 100 for 10^2, etc.).
9. Calculate to obtain the actual number of CFUs per milliliter of original undiluted sample.
10. Identification of the organism is performed using standard laboratory methods.

Interpretation

Threshold levels that define clinically significant cultures have been determined based on the intrinsic virulence of the organism and its occurrence as normal flora (Folkens et al. In press). In studies designed to evaluate the efficacy of antibacterial agents, these threshold values then are used to define clinically significant cultures and are minimum values required for enrollment of patients in a study. These also may serve as a reference point for comparison with subsequent cultures for determination of clinically significant effects in therapeutic trials.

Qualification

To qualify for inclusion in a clinical trial, the following parameters are used:

Equal to or Greater Than 1 CFU/mL:
Group A *Streptococcus*
Streptococcus pneumoniae
Neisseria spp
All gram-negative bacilli

Equal to or Greater Than 10 CFU/mL
Staphylococcus aureus
Moraxella catarrhalis
Streptococcus—alpha-hemolytic
Micrococcus sp

Equal to or Greater Than 100 CFU/mL
Staphylococcus epidermidis
Bacillus spp

Equal to or Greater Than 1000 CFU/mL
Corynebacterium spp
Results
Posttreatment cultures are then enumerated and organisms identified as de-
scribed earlier and can be interpreted by the following parameters suggested
by Folkens (in press):

Eradicated: numbers originally above threshold are reduced to zero
Significant reduction: decreased in number below threshold
Persistence: reduced in number but not below threshold
Proliferated: numbers originally above threshold are increased
Emergence: appearance of new organisms above threshold levels that were
not present in the original cultures

REFERENCES

Cagle GD, Abshire RL: Quantitative ocular bacteriology: A method for the enumera-
tion and identification of bacteria from the skin-lash margin and conjunctiva. Invest
Ophthalmol 1981;20:751–757.

Folkens AT, Schlech BA, Cupp GA, Wilmer Z: Quantitative ocular bacteriology. In Tabbara KF, Hyndiuk RA (eds.): Infections of the eye. 2nd Edition. Boston: Little,
Brown, (In press).

Antimicrobial Sensitivity Tests and Interpretation

8

Standardized disk diffusion techniques should be used for antibiotic susceptibility testing of bacteria. Results can be made available quickly, and disk diffusion testing allows greater flexibility in altering the choices of antimicrobial agents to be tested than do the automated or semiautomated systems. The ophthalmologist and microbiologist should be aware, however, that results of disk diffusion susceptibility tests relate to levels of drug achievable in serum and do not relate directly to the concentration of drug produced in the preocular tear film and ocular tissues by standard routes of administration. Estimating the minimal inhibitory concentrations of antibiotics may provide more useful information to the ophthalmologist than simply labeling an isolate as susceptible or resistant. The panel of antimicrobial agents to be tested should be chosen based on the relative susceptibility of the organism and in consideration of the pharmacy's formulary in each institution.

The value of antifungal susceptibility testing for therapy of ocular fungal infections has not been established. These procedures are available in some reference laboratories. The broth dilution method is the preferred technique for susceptibility testing of ocular yeasts and filamentous organisms. Determination should include the six antifungal agents of potential value in ocular infections: amphotericin B, natamycin (pimaricin), flucytosine, clotrimazole, miconazole, and ketoconazole.

8.1 DEFINITION OF SUSCEPTIBILITIES

Susceptible: An infection caused by the strain tests may be appropriately treated with the antimicrobic and dosages recommended for that type of infection and infecting species unless otherwise contraindicated.

Resistant: Strains that are not completely inhibited within the usual therapeutic dose range.

Intermediate: Includes strains that may respond to concentrations attainable by a usually high dosage or in areas where the antimicrobic is concentrated.

Minimal Inhibitory Concentration (MIC): The lowest concentration of antimicrobic that shows no visible growth.

Minimal Lethal Concentration (MLC) or Minimal Bactericidal Concentration (MBC): The lowest concentration of an antimicrobic that will kill all but a minimal defined proportion of viable organisms after incubation for a fixed time under a given set of conditions (99.9% lethal).

Persisters: A few (usually less than 0.1%), presumably metabolically inactive, organisms within a population that may survive the activity of a bactericidal antimicrobic. (Most apparent with beta-lactam antimicrobics).

Tolerance: The existence of an MLC-to-MIC ratio of 32 or greater after 24 hours of incubation. It is an unstable trait that can gradually be lost during storage.

Synergism: When the effect observed with the combination is greater than the sum of the effects observed using the two drugs independently.

8.2 STANDARDIZED DISK SUSCEPTIBILITY TESTS

Quantitative methods that require the measurement of zone sizes give the most precise estimates of antibiotic susceptibilities. The following outline describes such a procedure. Minor variations from this procedure may be used if the resulting procedure is standardized according to the results obtained in the laboratory from adequate studies with control cultures.

A. PREPARATION OF CULTURE MEDIUM AND PLATES

1. Melt previously prepared and sterilized Mueller-Hinton agar at medium heat and then cool to 45° to 50°C.
2. For the purpose of testing certain fastidious organisms such as streptococci and *Haemophilus spp*, 5% defibrinated horse or sheep blood may be added to the medium, which may be chocolatized when indicated.
3. To prepare the plates, pour the melted medium into petri dishes on a level surface to a depth of 4 mm.
4. Let the medium solidify and allow to stand long enough for excess moisture to evaporate. (For this purpose plates may be placed in an incubator at 35° to 37°C for 15 to 30 minutes or allowed to stand somewhat longer at room temperature). There should be no moisture droplets on the surface of the

medium or on the petri dish covers. The pH of the solidified medium should be 7.2 to 7.4. Satisfactory plates may be used immediately or refrigerated. Plates may be used as long as the surface is moist and there is no sign of deterioration.

NOTE: Commercially prepared agar plates meeting the above specifications may be used.

B. PREPARATION OF INOCULUM

1. Select four or five similar colonies.
2. Transfer these colonies (obtained by touching the top of each colony carefully with a wire loop) to a test tube containing approximately 5 mm of a suitable liquid medium such as soybean-casein digest broth, United States Pharmacopeia (U.S.P.), or tryptic soy broth.
3. Incubate the tube at 35° to 37°C long enough (2 to 8 hours) to produce an organism suspension with moderate cloudiness. At that point the inoculum density of the suspension should be controlled by diluting it, or a portion of it, with sterile saline to obtain a turbidity equivalent to that of a freshly prepared turbidity standard obtained by adding 0.5 mL of 1.175% barium chloride dehydrate ($BaCl_2.2H_2O$) solution to 99.5 mL 0.36 N (1%) sulfuric acid. Other suitable methods for standardizing inoculum density may be used; for example, a photometric method. In some cases it may be possible to get an adequate inoculum density in the tube even without incubation.

NOTE: Inoculum density should not exceed that of the standard. Undiluted overnight broth cultures should never be used for streaking plates.

C. INOCULATING THE PLATES

1. Dip a sterile cotton swab on a wooden applicator into the properly diluted inoculum. Remove excess inoculum from the swab by rotating it several times with firm pressure on the inside wall of the test tube above the fluid level.
2. Streak the swab over the entire sterile agar surface of the plate. Streaking successively in three different directions is recommended to obtain an even inoculum.
3. Replace the plate top and allow the inoculum to dry for 3 to 5 minutes.
4. Place the susceptibility disk on the inoculated agar surface with sterile forceps, or with a needle tip flamed and cooled between each use, gently press down each disk to insure even contact. Space the disk evenly so that they are no closer than 10 to 15 mL to the edge of the petri dish and sufficiently separated from each other to avoid overlapping zones of inhibition. (Spacing may be accomplished by using a disk dispenser or by putting the plate over a pattern to guide the placement of disk.) Within 30 minutes, place the plate in an incubator under aerobic conditions at a constant temperature in the range of 35° to 37°C. Fastidious organisms such as *Neisseriae,* which

may be affected by adverse atmospheric conditions, can be placed into a CO_2 incubator.

5. Read the plate after overnight incubation or, if rapid results are desired, the diameters of the zone of inhibition may be readable after 6 to 8 hours' incubation. In the latter case, the results should be confirmed by also reading the results after overnight incubation.

NOTE: Microbial growth on the plate should be just or almost confluent. If only isolated colonies are present, the inoculum was too light and the test should be repeated. If the growth near the disk is thick and double zones are seen, the inoculum was probably too heavy and this should be repeated.

D. READING THE PLATES

Measure and record the diameter of each zone (including the diameter of the disk) to the closest millimeter, reading to the point of complete inhibition as judged by the unaided eye. Preferably, read from the underside of the plate without removing the cover, using a calipers, ruler, transparent plastic gauge, or similar device. A mechanical zone reader may be used. If blood agar is used, measure the zones from the surface with the cover removed from the plate.

REFERENCES

Brinser JH: Practical ocular microbiology course 557. 1984. Department of Ophthalmology, College of Medicine, University of South Florida.

E. INTERPRETATION OF ZONE SIZES

1. Interpret the susceptibility according to the tables from the manufacturer's insert or statistical evaluations recommended by an outside quality control source. Ranges must be updated, and new antibiotics vary in susceptibility and availability within the generic drugs.
2. Staphylococci exhibiting resistance to the penicillinase-resistant penicillin class disks should be reported as resistant to cephalosporin-class antibiotics. The 30-μg cephalothin disk cannot be relied on to detect resistance of methicillin-resistant staphylococci to cephalosporin-class antibiotics.
3. The clindamycin disk is used for testing susceptibility to both clindamycin and lincomycin.
4. Colistin and polymyxin B diffuse poorly in agar, and the accuracy of the diffusion method is less than with other antibiotics. Resistance is always significant, but when treatment of systemic infections caused by susceptible strains is considered, it is wise to confirm the results of a diffusion test with a dilution method.
5. The methicillin disk is used for testing susceptibility to all penicillinase-resistant (beta-lactam) penicillins; that is, methicillin, cloxacillin, dicloxacillin, oxacillin, and nafcillin.

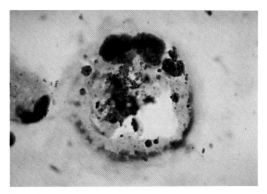

Plate 1
Macrophage cell in phacoanaphylactic endophthalmitis can engulf lens and iris. Megalomelanin
granules and piece of lens can be seen within the
cell. Giemsa stain, 1,000× magnification.

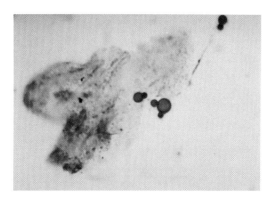

Plate 2
Yeast Malassezia furfur *can be seen in lid scrapings
but is generally not retrieved in culture. Giemsa
stain, 1,000× magnification.*

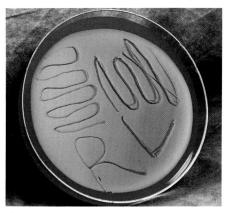

Plate 3
Inoculation streaks indicated for right (R),
left (L) eyelids and vertical and horizontal
serpentine streaks for respective conjunctivae.

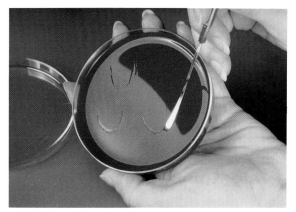

Plate 4
Multiple C-shapes are streaked onto the agars to indicate
cornea scrapings obtained by the ophthalmologist.

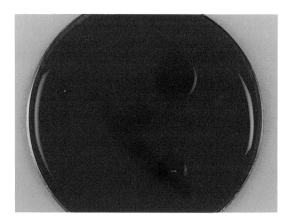

Plate 5
Fluids from sterile sources are inoculated in the center of the plate without
further manipulation, to avoid contamination.

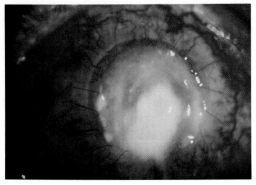

Plate 6
Fungal keratitis and secondary endophthalmitis resulting from contaminated donor material in post–penetrating keratoplasty surgery.

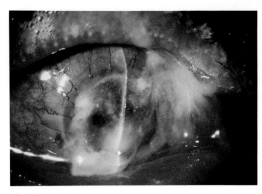

Plate 7
Clinical picture of patient suffering from post-PKP fungal endophthalmitis infection from contaminated donor tissue.

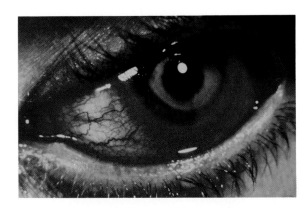

Plate 8
Characteristic ring form keratitis in Acanthamoeba *parasitemia. Courtesy of Frederick A. Jacobiec, M.D., Armed Forces Institute of Pathology, Washington, DC.*

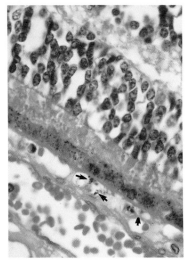

Plate 9
Hematoxylin and eosin–stained slide of malarial parasites in the ocular tissue. Courtesy of Robert Nalbandian, M.D., and Ahmed Hidayat, M.D., A.F.I.P., Washington, DC, reprinted by permission of Ophthalmology. *(1993; 100:1183–6).*

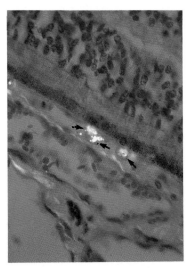

Plate 10
Birefringence of malarial pigment using polarized light. Courtesy of Robert Nalbandian, M.D., and Ahmed Hidayat, M.D., A.F.I.P., Washington, DC, reprinted by permission of Ophthalmology. *(1993; 100:1183–6).*

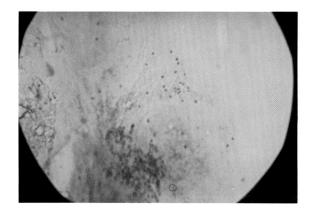

Plate 11
Many small gram-negative coccobacilli significant in Haemophilus influenzae conjunctivitis *in children. Gram stain, 1,000× magnification.*

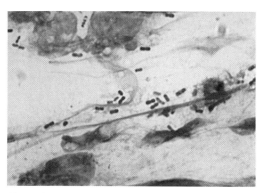

Plate 12
Moraxella spp *are frequently isolated in corneal infections and exhibit "diplobacilli" or characteristic boxcar shape. Gram stain, 1,000× magnification.*

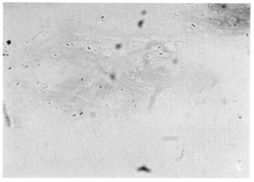

Plate 13
Streptococcus pneumoniae *may contain a capsule or other property of a mucopolysaccharide wall that causes them to decolorize easily and to appear gram-negative on occasion. A halo or capsule is seen against the cellular background. Gram stain, 1,000× magnification.*

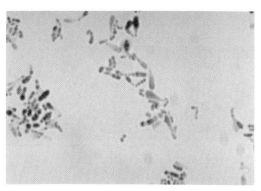

Plate 14
Bacteroides spp *are gram-negative anaerobes that exhibit club-shaped appearance and irregular staining properties. Gram stain, 1,000× magnification.*

Plate 15
Fungi may be present that do not stain at all, but their tree-formation shape can be detected against the cellular background and restained by another method for confirmation. Gram stain, 1,000× magnification.

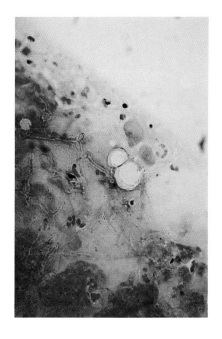

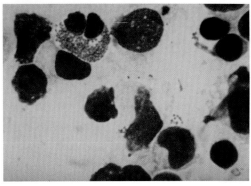

Plate 16
Mixed cells that may be seen in Giemsa-stained smears: eosinophil, lymphocyte, polymorphonuclear neutrophil, epithelial cells. Giemsa stain, 1,000× magnification.

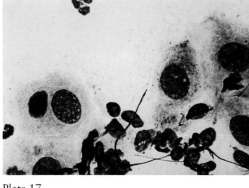

Plate 17
Inclusion (or chlamydial) conjunctivitis contains characteristic inclusions; elementary bodies can be seen outside the cell as it ruptures. Giemsa stain, 1,000× magnification.

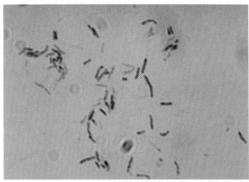

Plate 18
Mycobacterium tuberculosis *from corneal scraping stains acid-fast and often appears to bend in the middle. Kinyoun stain, 1,000× magnification.*

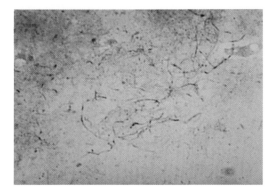

Plate 19
Actinomycetes *stain acid-fast; crushed granules from tissue may have filamentous branching rods with a beaded appearance. Ziehl-Neelsen stain, 1,000× magnification.*

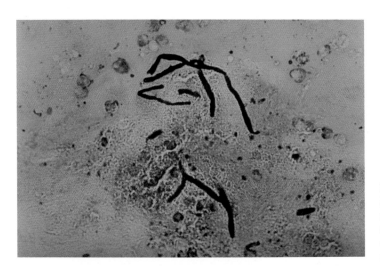

Plate 20
Dichotomous branching hyphae of Aspergillus flavus *from a clinical case of mycotic keratitis. Grocott-Gomori Methanamine silver (GMS) stain, 100× magnification.*

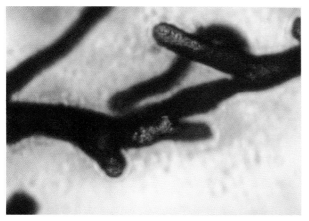

Plate 21
Fusarium solani *GMS-stained hyphae viewed with higher magnification show silver deposits and characteristic staining properties of fungi. Grocott-Gomori Methenamine silver stain, 1,000× magnification.*

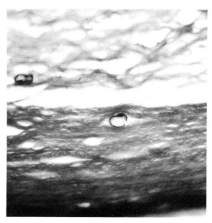

Plate 22
Acanthamoeba spp *cell walls stain silver-gray and can be seen deep in the corneal tissue. GMS stain, 500× magnification. Courtesy of Ahmed Hidayat, M.D., Department of Ophthalmic Pathology, AFIP, Washington, DC.*

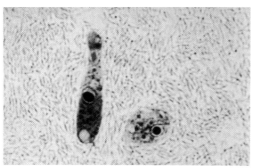

Plate 23
Hematoxylin & eosin–stained cyst and trophozoite from acanthamoebic keratitis. 50× magnification. Courtesy of Ahmed Hidayat, M.D., Department of Ophthalmic Pathology, AFIP, Washington, DC.

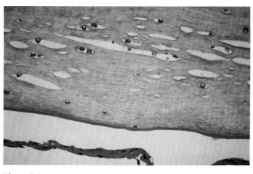

Plate 24
Hematoxylin & eosin–stained tissue showing cysts of Acanthamoeba spp *deep in the stromal layers of a keratoplasty tissue. Courtesy of Ahmed Hidayat, M.D., Department of Ophthalmic Pathology, Washington, DC.*

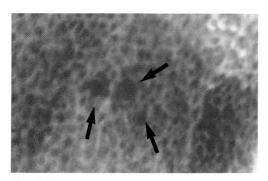

Plate 25
Goblet cells stain intensely pink in a sheet of conjunctival epithelium with mild scarring, obtained by impression cytology filter papers that have been stained.

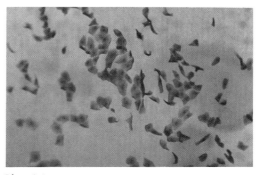

Plate 26
Abscence of goblet cells and excessive keratinization is seen in patients with various dry eye disorders or inactive trachoma by impression cytology methods.

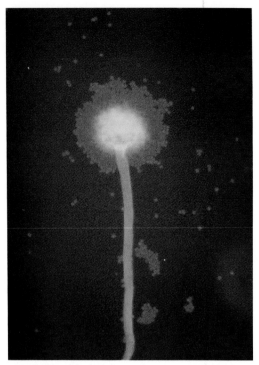

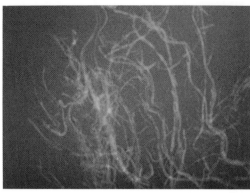

Plate 28
Apple-green fluorescence of hyphae may wane as hyphae ages, as seen on parts of these nonseptate hyphae from a clinical case of diabetic fungal endophthalmitis. Calcofluor white stain, 500× magnification.

Plate 27
Aspergillus flavus *from culture growth of cornea fluoresce brightly and appear red and orange because of the filter used. Calcofluor white stain, 500× magnification.*

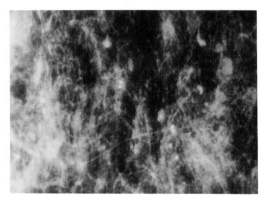

Plate 29
Yeast from Candida albicans *stain red and appear small at lower magnification and may be used as a positive control. Acridine orange stain, 400× magnification.*

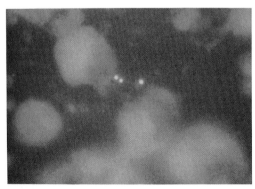

Plate 30
Elementary bodies fluoresce apple-green amidst counterstained epithelial cells. Microtrak monoclonal antibody DFA, 1,000× magnification.

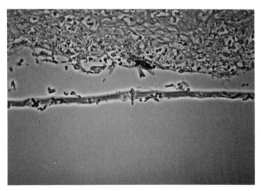

Plate 31
Hyphae in tissue along Descemet's membrane by phase microscopy, which may be performed on unstained tissue. 400× magnification.

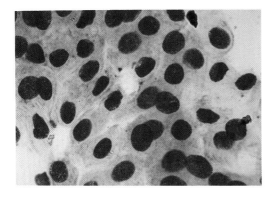

Plate 32
A Giemsa-stained conjunctival scraping showing normal epithelial cells. Note that the cells are grouped in sheets and are uniform in size and staining characteristics.

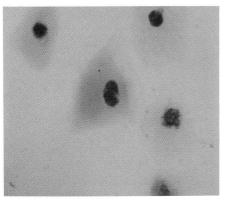

Plate 33
Keratinized epithelial cells seen in a conjunctival scraping from a patient with keratoconjunctivitis sicca. Note the pyknotic nuclei and pink-colored cytoplasm of these cells. Giemsa stain.

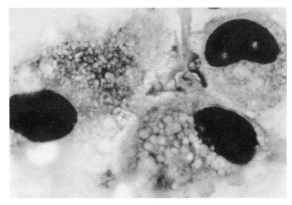

Plate 34
Abnormal epithelial cells in a scraping from a patient with a small irregular mass on the bulbar conjunctiva. The Giemsa-stained cells have irregular nuclei and show vacuolization of the cytoplasm. A biopsy of the mass later proved it to be a squamous cell carcinoma.

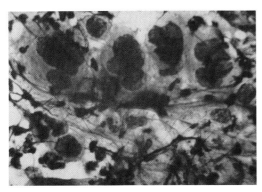

Plate 35
Multinucleated epithelial cells seen in a conjunctival scraping from a patient with primary herpes simplex keratoconjunctivitis. Giemsa stain.

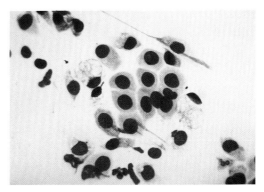

Plate 36
A Giemsa-stained smear showing goblet cells interspersed among normal epithelial cells in a patient with keratoconjunctivitis sicca. Goblet cells are distinguished by their eccentric nucleus and pink-staining mucoid material in the cytoplasm.

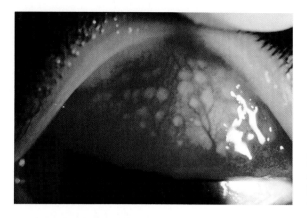

Plate 37
Moderate inflammation of the upper tarsal conjunctiva seen in a 10-year-old boy with trachoma.

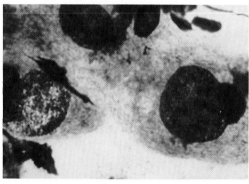

Plate 38
A Giemsa-stained smear from a patient with trachoma showing one epithelial cell with an early inclusion that "caps" the nucleus and another epithelial cell with a more advanced inclusion in which almost the entire cytoplasm is filled with elementary bodies.

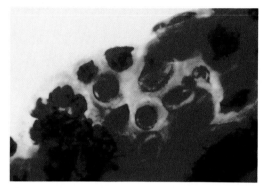

Plate 39
A Papanicolaou-stained scraping from a patient with herpes simplex keratitis. Intranuclear inclusions are observed in many cells and are detected by condensed nuclear chromatin with surrounding clear halo. Note that intranuclear inclusions are usually difficult to demonstrate in clinical specimens.

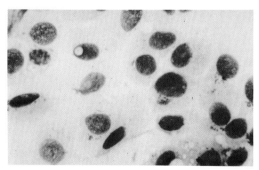

Plate 40
A Giemsa-stained smear from a patient with darkly pigmented skin, showing the presence of melanin granules in the epithelial cells. Melanin granules may resemble Chlamydia inclusions but are distinguished by their greenish-black stain and their presence in almost every cell in the scraping.

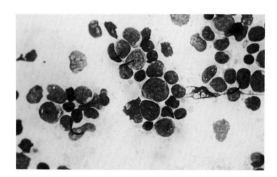

Plate 41
A conjunctival scraping from a patient with epidemic keratoconjunctivitis showing a mononuclear cell response typical of viral infections. Both large and small lymphocytes are seen, as well as normal epithelial cells. Giemsa stain.

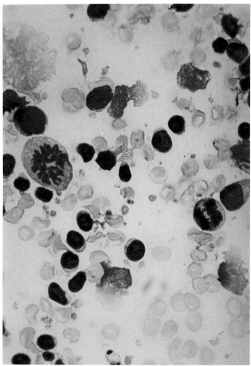

Plate 42
A Giemsa-stained scraping from a patient with severe trachoma, showing mitotic figures indicative of dividing lymphocytes in active inflammation.

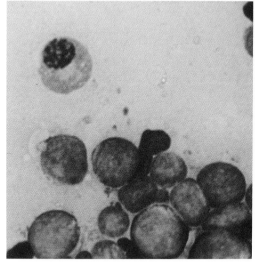

Plate 43
A Giemsa-stained conjunctival scraping from a patient with active trachoma, showing many blast cells with large, pale-staining nuclei and a plasma cell with an eccentric nucleus and adjacent clear area in the abundant cytoplasm.

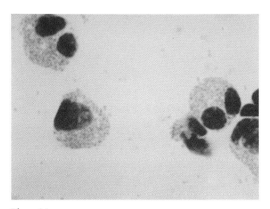

Plate 44
Eosinophils and some free eosinophilic granules are seen in this Giemsa-stained scraping from the upper tarsal conjunctiva of a patient with vernal conjunctivitis.

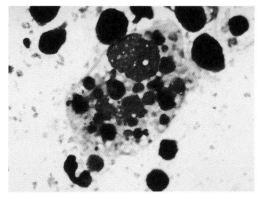

Plate 45
A Giemsa-stained smear from a trachoma patient showing Leber cells. Leber cells are large macrophages with abundant cellular debris in the cytoplasm.

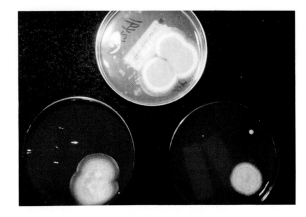

Plate 46
Hyphae present on all agars from C-streak areas in a case of Aspergillus flavus *keratitis in less than 48 hours.*

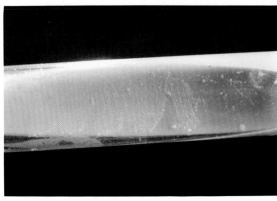

Plate 47
Lowenstein-Jensen media with grainy heavy growth of Mycobacterium tuberculosis *from direct inoculation of a corneal scraping.*

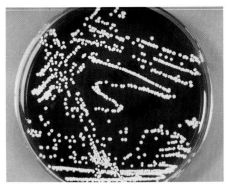

Plate 48
Blood agar incubated anaerobically from actinomycosis in clinical canaliculitis obtained from lacrimal fluid. Colonies may glisten or pit the agar and may be difficult to pry loose.

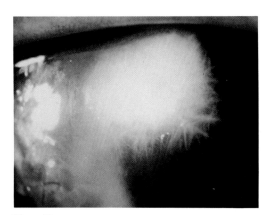

Plate 49
Chronic infectious crystalline keratopathy caused by alpha-streptococci (at high magnification) in a corneal transplant after treatment with topical corticosteroids for suspected graft reaction.

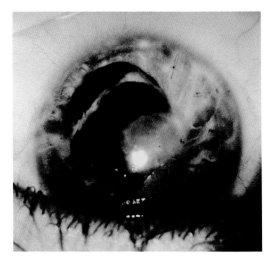

Plate 50
Complete resolution of disease after aggressive long-term therapy with topical ciprofloxacin alone.

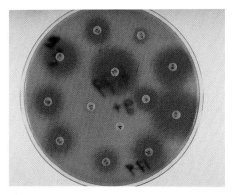

Plate 51
Antibiotic sensitivity disk diffusion tests run concurrently with test disk for preliminary identification of alpha- or beta-streptococci.

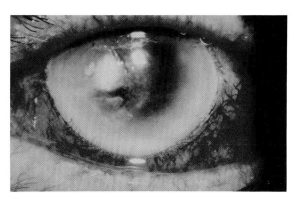

Plate 52
Classical Pseudomonas spp *ulcer with white infiltrate and diffuse epithelial haze after aphakic contact lens wear.*

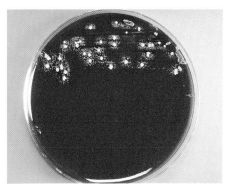

Plate 53
Colonies of Haemophilus influenzae *may satellite colonies of* Staphylococcus spp *on blood agar.*

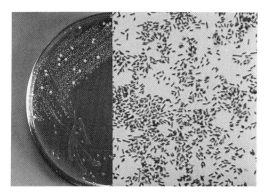

Plate 54
Haemophilus spp *grow well on chocolate agar and organisms appear small and coccobacillary when Gram stained, 1,000× magnification.*

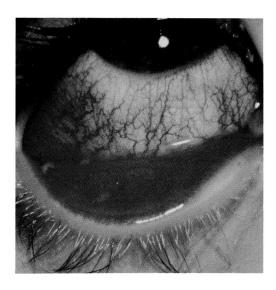

Plate 55
Clinical cases of conjunctivitis caused by Haemophilus influenzae *are common in young children and easily spread in the preschool environment.*

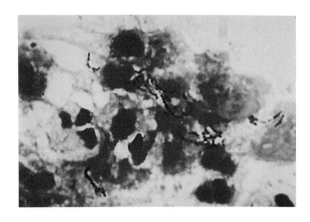

Plate 56
Gram-positive cocci in chains typical of group A streptococcal corneal ulcers from clinical scraping.

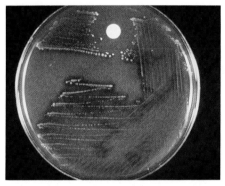

Plate 57
Preliminary identification of group A streptococci is facilitated by the bacitracin disk test on subculture. Note zone of sensitivity.

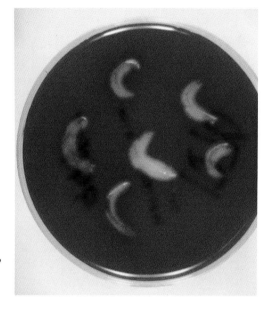

Plate 58
Green (alpha) or partial hemolysis on sheep blood agar characteristic of Streptococcus pneumoniae.

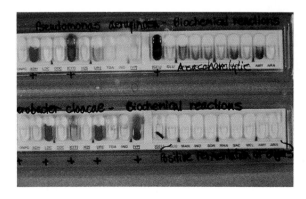

Plate 59
Pseudomonas aeruginosa *does not use many carbohydrates in API tests, but is generally GEL and CIT and ADH positive, as shown here in comparison with coliform bacteria reactions.*

6. Staphylococci exhibiting resistance to the beta-lactamase–resistant penicillin class discs such as methicillin should be reported as resistant to cephalosporin-class antibiotics. The 30-µg cephalothin disk cannot be relied on to detect resistance of methicillin-resistant staphylococci to cephalosporin-class antibiotics.

7. The oleandomycin disk is used for testing susceptibility to oleandomycin and troleandomycin.

8. The penicillin G disk is used for testing susceptibility to all penicillinase-susceptible except ampicillin and carbenicillin; that is, penicillin G, phenoxymethyl penicillin, and phenethicillin.

9. This category includes some organisms such as enterococci and gram-negative bacilli that may cause systemic infections treatable with high doses of penicillin G. Such organisms should only be reported susceptible to penicillin G and not to phenoxymethyl penicillin or phenethicillin.

10. Ciprofloxacin disks may be used for O-floxacin susceptibility, but the reverse has not been evaluated. Very high concentrations of the quinolones, especially ciprofloxacin and ofloxacin, may be achieved in ocular tissue after topical administration. Most of the pharmakokinetic studies have been done with ciprofloxacin. McDermott et al. (1993) demonstrated intra-corneal levels of ciprofloxacin of 5.28 ± 3.4 µg/g tissue after aggressive topical administration of ciprofloxacin (every 15 minutes for 1 hour then every hour for 10 hours) in patients (with intact epithelium) before penetrating keratoplasty. Penetration into the aqueous humor after a single systemic dose in patients undergoing ocular surgery is in the range of 20% for ofloxacin and approximately 15% for ciprofloxacin. Clinically the quinolones may be highly effective even in streptococcal corneal infections, because concentrations significantly above their MICs may be easily achieved in corneal infection when aggressive topical treatment is given. Aggressive topical ciprofloxacin therapy alone has cured cases of difficult to treat "chronic" infectious crystalline keratopathy caused by alpha-hemolytic *Streptococcus*, as shown in Plate 49 before and Plate 50 after treatment.

Traditional antibiotic susceptibility disk testing for alpha-streptococcus, including pneumococcus, may include the optochin disk and bacitracin disk tests added to rule out *S. pneumoniae*, and beta-hemolytic Group A streptococci (described in Chapter 9), as shown in Plate 51. Typical sensitivity zones of *Pseudomonas aeruginosa* can be seen in Figure 8.1.

Reference organisms and stock cultures

1. Maintain stock cultures of *Staphylococcus aureus* (ATCC 25923) and *Escherichia coli* (ATCC 25922).

2. Test these reference organisms daily using antibiotic disk representative of those to be used in the testing of clinical isolates.

3. The individual values of zone sizes for the control organisms can be expected to fall in the ranges indicated in the table contained in manufacturer's insert accompanying commercial antibiotic disks from suppliers such as BBL.

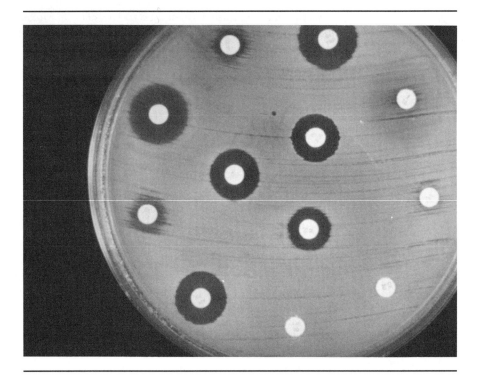

Figure 8.1
Standardized disk susceptibility tests for Pseudomonas aeruginosa.

BIBLIOGRAPHY

ASM-2 performance standards for antimicrobial disc susceptibility tests, 2nd Edition. Villanova, PA: National Committee for Clinical Laboratory Standards, 1992.

Barza M: Treatment of eye infections. In Hooper DC, Wolfson JS (eds.): Quinolone antimicrobial agents. Washington, DC: American Society for Microbiology, 1993.

McDermott ML, Tran TD, Cowden JW, Bugge CJL: Corneal stromal penetration of topical ciprofloxacin in humans. Ophthalmology 1993;100:197–200.

Methods for dilution: Antimicrobial susceptibility tests for bacteria that grow aerobically, approved standard: M7-A3, 3rd Edition. Villanova, PA: National Committee for Clinical Laboratory Standards, 1993.

8.3 ANTIBIOTICS OF CHOICE

Staphylococcus aureus, beta-lactamase positive (85%) and negative (15%)
Penicillin is the drug of choice for rarely encountered negative isolates; Ampicillin, carbenicillin, and the newer extended-spectrum penicillins (piperacillin) are ineffective against beta-lactamase–positive isolates. The drug of first choice is oxacillin or other beta-lactamase–resistant penicillins. First-generation cephalosporins are drugs of choice for both beta-

lactamase–positive and beta-lactamase–negative infections in allergic patients. Second-generation cephalosporins (cefoxitin) and third-generation cephalosporins (cefotaxime, etc.) are never indicated, but are usually effective. Vancomycin is effective for the very rare methicillin-resistant isolates. Clindamycin is reported to be effective in orthopedic infections, and erythromycin has efficacy in treating minor skin infections. Ciprofloxacin and other quinolones may not be clinically effective, but aggressive therapy using topical ciprofloxacin alone for bacterial keratitis has shown good results in clinical cases in our experience.

Staphylococcus saprophyticus
See recommendations for *S. aureus*.

Staphylococcus epidermidis
Organism shows a high rate of resistance to beta-lactamase–resistant penicillins and to cephalosporins. Vancomycin is the drug of choice for significant infections.

Enterococcus
Relatively resistant organism. In significant soft tissue infections, a combination of ampicillin (vancomycin if patient is penicillin allergic) plus gentamicin is appropriate. High-level aminoglycoside sensitivity testing and beta-lactamase testing should be done on isolates from blood cultures or serious intraocular infections. Isolates resistant to high levels (i.e., >2000 μg/mL) of gentamicin may be sensitive to streptomycin, and vice versa. The rarely encountered beta-lactamase–positive enterococci resist both gentamicin and streptomycin, but can be treated with ampicillin/sulbactam.

Escherichia coli
Klebsiella
Proteus mirabilis
These isolates are usually sensitive to cefazolin. *Escherichia coli* and *Proteus mirabilis* are occasionally resistant to ampicillin and amoxicillin. *Klebsiella* is resistant to ampicillin. Sensitivity data can be relied on. For the rare isolates that are resistant to cefazolin or the more unusual isolates that have MICs of 8 μg/mL, it is appropriate to consider the use of cefoxitin or a third-generation cephalosporin if the latter have more favorable MICs.
At least for serious ocular infections involving other tissues and septicemia, initial treatment should include gentamicin until the patient is well on the way to recovery. Many experts prefer to add an extended-spectrum penicillin or cephalosporin because of presumed, but not proven synergistic effect.

STREPTOCOCCI (*S. pneumoniae, S. bovis, Groups A through G, especially viridans,* etc.)
Very sensitive to penicillin, ampicillin, first-generation cephalosporins, erythromycin, clindamycin, and vancomycin. Third-generation cephalosporins and extended-spectrum penicillins are never indicated, but are effective. Resistant to tetracyclines, aminoglycosides, aztreonam, ciprofloxacin, and other quinolones.

RESISTANT GRAM-NEGATIVE ROD. Includes all species of *Enterobacter Serratia, Proteus vulgaris, Providencia, Citrobacter,* etc.
Sensitivity data for cephalosporins are sometimes (approximately 10%) unreliable in predicting clinical success. Gentamicin should be used, perhaps

Agent	Gram-positive organisms	Gram-negative cocci	Gram-negative rods	Pseudomonas aeruginosa
Penicillins	+	+	+	
Carbenicillin			+	+
Nafcillin, Oxacillin, or Methicillin	+			
Penicillin G	+	+		
Bacitracin	+			
Cephalosporin	+	+		
Chloramphenicol	+	+	+	
Clindamycin	+			
Erythromycin	+	+		
Vancomycin	+			
Fucidin	+			
Minocycline	+	+	+	
Quinolones (CiproFloxacin)	+	+	+	+
Amikacin			+	+
Gentamicin	+		+	+
Neomycin	+		+	+
Tobramycin	+		+	+
Polymyxin B			+	+
Tetracycline	+	+	+	

with an extended-spectrum penicillin or cephalosporin. It is appropriate to use trimethoprim/sulfamethoxazole or ciprofloxacin if the organism tests sensitive *in vitro* for infections that are not serious.

Pseudomonas

Despite favorable sensitivity data, monotherapy with extended-spectrum penicillins or any cephalosporin is likely to be ineffective. Always use gentamicin, tobramycin, or amikacin. Many experts add carbenicillin or ceftazidime for synergy in serious infections. Topical therapy with ciprofloxacin is generally effective, as described previously. Classical *Pseudomonas* corneal ulcers exhibit a white infiltrate with diffuse epithelial haze, as shown in Plate 52, after aphakic contact lens wear.

Bacteroides fragilis

Clindamycin or metronidazole should be used in the therapy or prophylaxis of infections caused by these agents. Cefoxitin is more active against these bacteria than are third-generation cephalosporins, but sensitivity to cefoxitin, third-generation cephalosporins, and extended-spectrum penicillins is less predictable. Aztreonam, ciprofloxacin, and other quinolones are not generally effective.

OTHER ANAEROBES

Penicillin, first-generation cephalosporins, and clindamycin are all equally effective and drugs of choice. Metronidazole is effective against *Bacteroides*. Its efficacy against anaerobic streptococci is controversial. *Clostridium difficile* is usually treated with oral vancomycin or oral metronidazole. Aztreonam, ciprofloxacin, and other quinolones are not effective.

Neisseria gonorrhoeae, beta-lactamase–positive (<1%) or –negative (99%)
Penicillin is the drug of choice for beta-lactamase–negative isolates. Infections caused by beta-lactamase–positive isolates or infections in allergic patients may be treated with ceftriaxone. Spectinomycin is effective, except for
treating pharyngeal gonorrhea. Tetracyclines are less effective alternatives.

The selection of antimicrobial agents for susceptibility testing of ocular isolates
is listed on page 112.

BIBLIOGRAPHY

Chambers HF: Methicillin-resistant staphylococci. Clin Microbiol Rev 1988;1:
173–186.
Eng RK, et al.: Inoculum effect of new beta lactam antibiotics on Pseudomonas aerugi-
nosa. Antimicrob Agents Chemother 1987;26:42–47.
Follath F: Clinical consequences of development of resistance to third generation
cephalosporins. Eur J Clin Microbiol 1987;6:446–450.
Gardner OA, Lorian V: Bacterial susceptibility to antibiotics remains virtually stable.
Antimicrob Newsl 1985;2:9–14.
Performance standards for antimicrobial disk susceptibility tests, approved standard:
M2–A5 with supplements. Villanova, PA: National Committee for Clinical Labora-
tory Standards, 1993.
Sanders C, Sanders W: Inducible beta-lactamases: Clinical and epidemiological impli-
cations for use of newer cephalosporins. Rev Infect Dis 1988;10:830–838.
Sanders C, Sanders W: Microbial resistance to newer generation beta lactam antibiotics:
Clinical and laboratory implications. J Infect Dis 1985;151:399–406.
Soriana F, et al.: In vivo significance of the inoculum effect of antibiotics on *E. coli.* J
Clin Microbiol Infect Dis 1988;7:410–412.
Thornsberry C: Methicillin resistant (heteroresistant) staphylococci. Antimicrob Newsl
1984;1:43–49.
Washington JA: Discrepancies between in vitro activity of and in vivo response to an-
timicrobial agents. Diagn Microbiol Infect Dis 1983;1:25–31.
Wegner D: Predictable antibiotic susceptibility, session 47, 1993. Northwest Sympo-
sium by the Pacific Area Resource Office of the National Laboratory Training Net-
work and Centers for Disease Control, 1993.
Weisblum B: Inducible beta lactamase in bacteria. Br Med Bull 1984;40:4753.

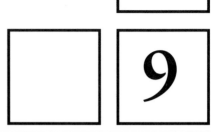

Identification Schemes for Common Isolates

9

Many laboratories employ automated systems of identification (Vitek, etc.). In smaller institutions, however, the Analytical Profile Index (API, bio Mérieux Vitek Inc, Hazelwood, MO) may still be used with a database of comparable biochemical reactions. The following is a guideline to preliminary and biochemical identification of common isolates in external eye disease.

9.1 PRELIMINARY IDENTIFICATION OF BACTERIAL ISOLATES

It is often necessary to perform spot testing on isolates to speed preliminary identification. This is very important because some gram-negative rods and staphylococcal or streptococcal infections can be very damaging in the eye. *Haemophilus* can often be seen satelliting *Staphylococcus* colonies if *Staphylococcus* is also present, as shown in Plate 53, and grows well on chocolate agar in Plate 54. The organisms are short, small, and occasionally coccobacilli or thin as in *H. aegyptius*. Most *Haemophilus* infections are caused by *H. influenzae*. This form of conjunctivitis is common in children and is easily treatable. A characteristic clinical picture is shown in Plate 55.

Beta-hemolytic *Streptococcus* group A appears gram positive in chains on initial smears from corneal scrapings, as shown in Plate 56, and clinically may present with a sterile hypopyon, as in Figure 9.1 corneal ulcer after an unknown foreign body injury. Beta-hemolysis is easily recognized on blood or chocolate agars, resulting in clear zones within the C-streaks, as seen in Figure 9.2 Identification of group A is substantiated by bacitracin disk sensitivity zone on sub-

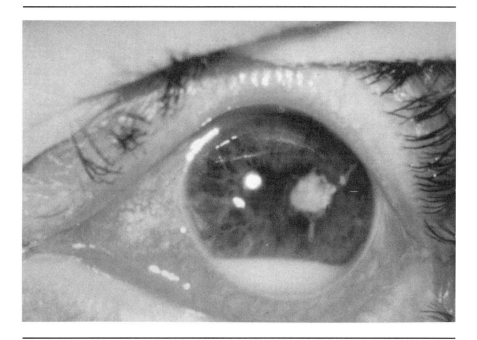

Figure 9.1
Clinical case of a corneal ulcer caused by beta-hemolytic streptococci with a sterile hypopyon after unknown foreign body injury.

culture as demonstrated in Plate 57 or by agglutination identification tests described later. Alpha-hemolysis (also referred to as partial hemolysis) appears as green zones seen in C-streaks of plate media in Plate 58. Diplococci characteristic of *Streptococcus pneumoniae* may demonstrate capsules, lancet shape, and appear in pairs in initial smears Gram stained from scrapings (Figure 9.3). *Pseudomonas aeruginosa* are very serious ocular infectious agents and may rapidly perforate the cornea with subsequent endophthalmitis. They appear as slender gram-negative rods in vitreous and aqueous fluids, as shown in Figure 9.4. These organisms are oxidase positive and asaccharolytic in biochemical reactions, but are often gelatin, arginine dihydrolase (ADH), and citrate positive compared with coliform bacteria, as seen in Plate 59. *Bacillus cereus* has recently become an important pathogen in fulminating panophthalmitis in intravenous drug users or foreign body injuries, as shown in clinical picture Figure 9.5, and it could be confused with clostridia if accompanied by intraocular gas or appearance in Gram-stained preparations as in Figure 9.6. Special isolation media is available commercially, but taxonomic differentiation should be done by a reference laboratory or Centers for Disease Control because there are hundreds of strains of this genera. *Neisseria gonorhoeae* conjunctivitis is very vision threatening and may invade and perforate the cornea, as shown in Figure 9.7, and may require rapid identification to facilitate proper treatment.

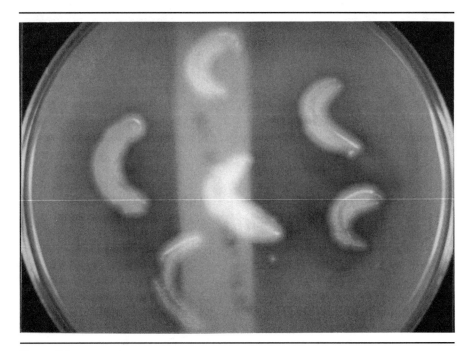

Figure 9.2
Clear (beta) hemolysis characteristic of group A streptococci on chocolate agar from a case of keratitis.

Materials and reagents

1. **Spot indole reagent.** (Paradimethylaminocinnamaldehyde). May be purchased from Remel Laboratories in Lenexa, Kansas. Store at 2° to 8°C.
2. **Rapid urea broth.** Obtain from Remel. Prepare according to directions and store in 0.5-mL aliquots in the freezer.
3. **L-phenylalanine.** Obtain from Sigma Chemical Company, St. Louis, Missouri. Make up as 1% solution in physiologic saline and store frozen in 0.5-mL aliquots. Some laboratories have been successful in storing it in a plastic bottle at room temperature, dispensing it as needed.
4. **Dry slide oxidase.** Store as directed. Difco Laboratories, Detroit, MI. Available from Remel and other distributors.
5. **Ornithine decarboxylase (ODC) strips.** Available from Key Scientific Products, Round Rock, Texas. Store at room temperature.
6. **PYR paper disks.** Obtain from Remel or other distributor. Store at 2° to 8°C.
7. **10% ferric chloride.** Obtain from Remel or PML Microbiologicals (Tagletin, Oregon). Store at 2° to 8°C.
8. **Hydrogen peroxide.** 3% for catalase testing. Obtain from any pharmacy. Store at 2° to 8°C.
9. **Bile solubility test reagent.** (10% deoxycholate, Remel) Store at 2° to 8°C.
10. *Staphylococcus aureus* **agglutination identification reagent** (BBL). Cefinase beta-lactamase disks. Store at 2° to 8°.

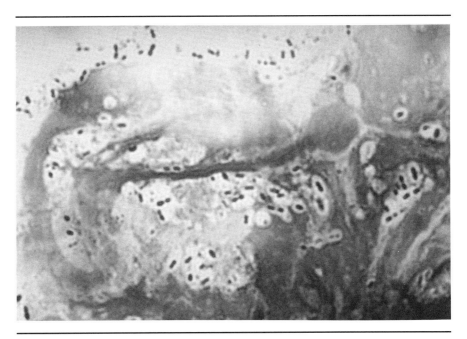

Figure 9.3
Gram-stained smear showing heavy presence of encapsulated, lancet-shaped pneumococcus from a case of bacterial keratitis.

11. **Novobiocin differentiation disks** (5 mcg). Obtain from Remel or Scott Laboratories. Store at 2° to 8°C.
12. **Group A Streptococci agglutination identification reagent.** Store as directed. Prepare according to manufacturer.

Follow manufacturer's instructions for preliminary spot tests and report as "**presumptive**" *Staphylococcus aureus*, Group A *Streptococcus*, *Pseudomonas*, etc.," based on expected results of these isolates until follow-up testing and complete biochemical tests are performed.

Preliminary identification of commonly isolated gram-negative bacilli
Rapid test protocols are described here; however, manufacturer's instructions should be adhered to for specifics.

1. Spot Indole Test
    a. Touch swab to moisten in broth media.
    b. Place 1 drop of spot reagent on the tip of a cotton swab. Touch swab to one or two colonies of the gram-negative organisms growing on blood, chocolate, or trypticase soy agar (cannot be performed from MacConkey, eosin-methylene blue, or selective media agar).

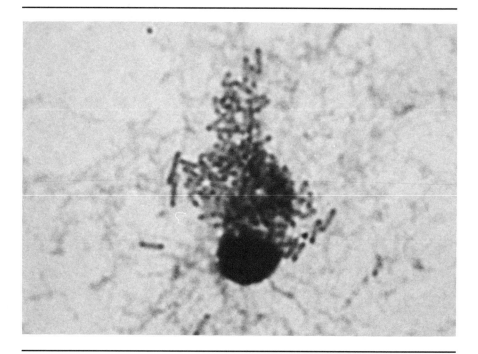

Figure 9.4
Vitreous specimen from a case of endophthalmitis had heavy gram-negative rods that were thin and sometimes showed spotty color if previously treated with antibiotics. Pseudomonas aeruginosa *isolated in later cultures.*

    c. Development of a blue color on swab within 60 seconds indicates a positive result. If there is no color change (swab remains yellow), the test is negative.

2. Rapid Urea Broth
    a. Remove a tube of broth from freezer and allow to thaw.
    b. Remove isolated colonies (3 or more) and inoculate the broth.
    c. Incubate at 35°C. Read at 30 minutes, 1 hour, and 90 minutes for the development of a pink color (positive test). Most urease-positive isolates will be detected in the first hour.
    d. If broth remains salmon pink colored, the test is negative.

3. Rapid Phenylalanine Deaminase (PDA) test
    a. Remove a tube of 1% L-phenylalanine from freezer and allow to thaw.
    b. Pick seven or eight well-isolated colonies of test organism and make a milky suspension.
    c. Incubate 1 hour at 34° to 37°C.
    d. Add 2 to 3 drops of ferric chloride and read immediately for the development of a green color, which indicates a positive test. If the tube remains the yellow color of the ferric chloride reagent, the organism is PDA negative.
    e. If unable to obtain seven or eight well-isolated colonies, incubate 90 minutes before adding the ferric chloride indicator reagent.

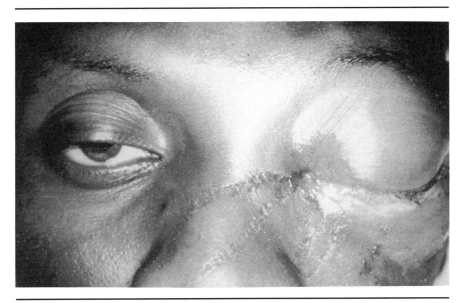

Figure 9.5
Bacillus cereus *panophthalmitis after an injury with a piece of metal produced gas evident in computed tomography scan and during surgery. Presumed clostridial clinically.*

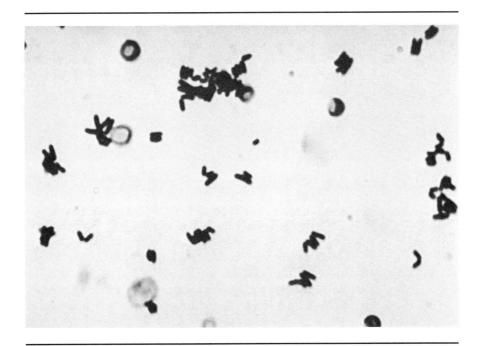

Figure 9.6
Gram-positive rods from Gram-stained vitreous and aqueous specimens from a fulminating panophthalmitis associated with intraocular gas proved to be Bacillus cereus *in culture examination.*

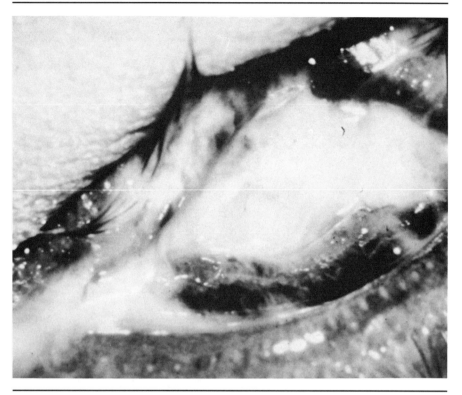

Figure 9.7
Severe gonococcal conjunctivitis and perforated corneal ulcer in an adult homosexual. Patient was placed on gentamicin for symptomatic conjunctivitis and progressed to perforation, which was treated by cyanoacrylate adhesion and resolved by aggressive topical therapy with ciprofloxacin.

4. Rapid Ornithine Decarboxylase (ODC) Test
    a. In a plastic, disposable screw cap test tube, place 1 mL fresh, reagent-grade distilled water.
    b. Pick four to eight well-isolated colonies of lactose-fermenting test organisms, and emulsify in the distilled water.
    c. Add an ODC test strip to the tube, cap, and incubate at 34° to 37°C for 2 hours. If suspension has a red tint, it is positive. If it is yellow, reincubate and observe periodically for an additional 2 hours.
    d. If it remains yellow at 4 hours, the organism is ODC negative.
5. Cytochrome Oxidase Test
    a. Open the Dry Slide Oxidase pouch and remove required number of slides.
    b. Fold the top of the pouch over once and seal tightly with a self-adhesive sticker (usually provided). Discard unused slides 1 week after the package is opened.
    c. Pick one or two colonies to be tested using a stick or plastic loop. **NOTE:** Using nichrome or other iron-containing devices may cause false-positive reactions.

d. Rub the organism directly onto a portion of a reaction area of the Dry Slide Oxidase. (Each reaction area can accommodate up to four tests). Development of a purple color within 20 seconds indicates a positive test. **NOTE:** Color development after 20 seconds should be disregarded. No color change is a negative test.

B. Rapid gram-negative test indications:

Organism type	Spot indole	Rapid urea	Ornithine decarboxylase (ODC)	Rapid PDA
Lactose Fermenter	Yes	If Spot Indole Negative	If Spot Indole Negative Discard if Urea Positive	No
Swarming, non–lactose fermenter	Yes	Yes	No	No
Oxidase-positive, nonswarming, non–lactose fermenter	No	No	No	No
Oxidase-negative nonswarming, non–lactose fermenter isolates.	Yes	Yes	No	Yes

C. Identification flow charts (Wegner, et al.)

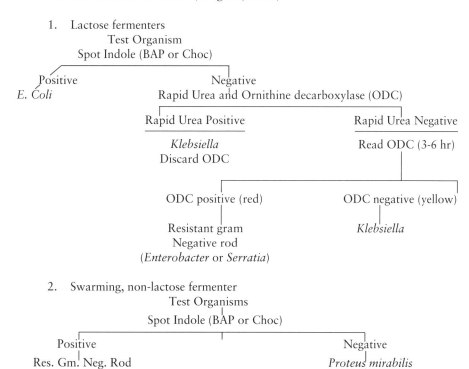

1. Lactose fermenters
   Test Organism
   Spot Indole (BAP or Choc)

   Positive → *E. Coli*
   Negative → Rapid Urea and Ornithine decarboxylase (ODC)

   Rapid Urea Positive → *Klebsiella* Discard ODC
   Rapid Urea Negative → Read ODC (3-6 hr)

   ODC positive (red) → Resistant gram Negative rod (*Enterobacter* or *Serratia*)
   ODC negative (yellow) → *Klebsiella*

2. Swarming, non-lactose fermenter
   Test Organisms
   Spot Indole (BAP or Choc)

   Positive → Res. Gm. Neg. Rod (*Proteus vulgaris*) Rapid urea negative
   Negative → *Proteus mirabilis* Rapid urea positive

3. Oxidase positive non–lactose-fermenters
    Because infection with oxidase-positive gram-negatives other than
    Pseudomonas is very rare, these may be reported as presumptive
    Pseudomonas, because antibiotic therapy is the same.
4. Oxidase-negative nonswarming, non–lactose-fermenters

Test Organsim
|
Spot Indole, PDA, Rapid Urea

Indole - Pos PDA - Pos Urea - Pos	Indole - Pos PDA - Pos Urea - Neg	Indole - Pos PDA - Neg Urea - Neg	Indole - Neg PDA - Neg Urea - Pos	Indole - Neg PDA - Pos Urea - Pos	Indole - Neg PDA - Neg Urea - Neg
Res. Grm. Neg. rod usually (*Morganella, Providencia*)	Res. Grm. Neg. rod usually (*Providencia stuartii*)	*E. Coli*	*Klebsiella*	*P. mirabilis*	Res. Grm. Neg. rod usually (*Enterobacter* and others)

Grouping of staphylococcal isolates

Test aerobically growing gram-positive cocci for catalase reaction by picking
one or two colonies and mixing with 1 drop of 3% hydrogen peroxide. If the
colonies bubble, this indicates the organism is catalase positive and belongs to
the staphylococci. Note that: (1) Dropping catalase reagent directly on colonies
on agar is not recommended because many common agars, such as sheep blood
agar, have catalase activity and can give false-positive reactions. (2) Gram-
negative inhibitory agars, such as phenethyl alcohol (PEA) or calcium nutrient
agar (CNA), may have staphylococcal isolates that test as catalase negative. If
an isolate on one of these plates morphologically resembles staphylococci but
gives a negative catalase test, subculture to a plain blood agar plate and retest
catalase the next day.

Differentiate *Staphylococcus aureus* from other staphylococci using an agglutination identification reagent. Proceed as directed by the package insert.
The tube coagulase test, performed as directed by microbiology textbooks, can
be used as a substitute or a backup method.

1. Report all reagent-positive or tube coagulase-positive isolates (negative
    control very important) as *Staphylococcus aureus.*
2. Report beta-lactamase result on all *Staphylococcus aureus,* using BBL (Cock-
    eysville, Maryland) Cefinase disks or other commercial beta-lactamase de-
    tection kits. If an isolate appears initially to be beta lactamase negative,
    incubate up to 30 minutes before calling it beta lactamase negative, because
    some isolates may possess only the inducible beta-lactamase enzyme.
3. **IMPORTANT:** Note that some *Staphylococcus aureus* isolates on CNA or
    PEA may be slightly inhibited, causing them to give false-negative Staphylo-
    coccal agglutination identification reagent, tube coagulase, or beta-lactamase
    results. If an isolate gives separate colonies only on PEA or CNA agar, re-
    sembles *Staphylococcus aureus,* but gives a negative agglutination identifica-

tion reagent reaction, tube coagulase, or beta-lactamase result, subculture to a plain blood agar plate and retest the next day.

4. Extremely young isolates of *Staphylococcus aureus* may give false-negative reactions on blood or other agars. Retest after an additional day's incubation if the colonies resemble those of *Staphylococcus aureus* or perfom tube coagulase test the same day.

5. Report agglutination identification reagent or tube coagulase–negative staphylococcal isolates as presumptive *Staphylococcus epidermidis*. No speciation beyond this is indicated, except for deep ocular culture isolates such as endophthalmitis.

Differentiate *Staphylococcus epidermidis* from *Staphylococcus saprophyticus* on patients who may have secondary complications such as positive blood cultures by doing Novobiocin sensitivity on staphylococcal agglutination identification reagent–negative (or tube coagulase–negative) isolates. Inoculate organism into a tube of sensitivity broth and incubate approximately 4 hours.

Adjust density with saline to that of a 0.5 MacFarland (Kirby-Bauer) turbidity standard. Make a lawn of organism on a blood agar plate by streaking with a cotton or dacron swab in three directions. Place a 5-µg novobiocin differentiation disk (which is different from the Kirby-Bauer sensitivity disk) on the plate and incubate overnight without CO_2.

Measure zone size the next day. If it is smaller than 16 mm, report as *S. saprophyticus*.

Identification flow chart

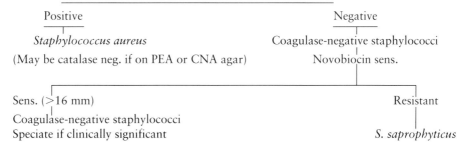

Grouping of aerobic streptococcal isolates:

A. Perform bacitracin sensitivity, optochin sensitivity, and agglutination according to package insert instructions supplied with manufacturer's commercial product.

B. Pyroglutamic acid-β-napthylamide hydrolysis (PYR reaction)
   1. Remove PYR disk from bottle, using forceps, and place on agar plate.
   2. Wet disk with 1 drop sterile water.
   3. Pick one to two colonies of organism to be tested and rub gently onto PYR disk.

4. Incubate at room temperature for 2 minutes.
5. Add 1 drop PYR reagent.
6. Read test at 1 minute. If test is positive, the disk will turn red. If test is negative, the disk will remain white or yellow.
7. Note the Group A beta-hemolytic streptococci and some staphylococci give positive reactions.

C. Flow chart for alpha-hemolytic streptococci from cultures of all sterile sites (e.g., cornea, vitreous) and naso/lacrimal or lower respiratory tract specimens. Do only on clinically significant isolates, as determined by Gram stain of original specimen.

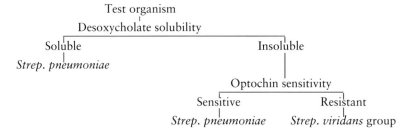

Flow Chart for Beta-Hemolytic Streptococci

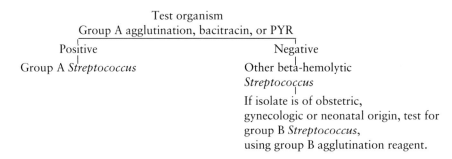

Flow chart for significant alpha and gamma (nonhemolytic) clinically significant isolates (see appropriate specimen culture procedure to determine if isolate is clinically significant and warrants procedure below).

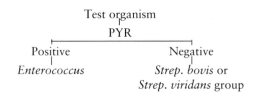

Further speciation of alpha- and gamma-hemolytic streptococci, beyond deciding if isolate is or is not an *Enterococcus*, is warranted if it is from a sterile source or if patient also has complications including positive blood culture with endocarditis. Use API *Streptococcus* strip or reference laboratory to do this. Different species of streptococci within the classical *Streptococcus viridans* group have different prognoses and vary in their degree of penicillin sensitivity.

Preliminary identification of other organisms
(Use commercial product or method(s) described below)

A. *Haemophilus*
   1. XV factor quad plates. Available from Remel (Lenexa, KS).
   2. Spot indole–positive isolates from lacrimal and conjunctival specimens whose Gram stain, colony morphology, and growth requirements match those of *Haemophilus* can be called *Haemophilus spp.*
   3. Innovative Diagnostics Rapid NH method (Atlanta, Georgia, Telephone 800-241-2926).
B. *Branhamella* and *Neisseria spp:* Use Innovative Diagnostics Systems Rapid NH method.
C. *Neisseria gonorrhoeae.*
   Use agglutination or a monoclonal antibody latex agglutination method to identify these. They work best with heavy, boiled suspensions of overnight subcultures of test isolates.
D. Anaerobes
   1. Because of the multiple antibiotic resistances of *Bacteroides*, report beta-lactamase–positive gram-negative bacilli, whose growth requirements and Gram stain morphology are consistent with *Bacteroides*, as *Bacteroides* species.
   2. Use commercially available anaerobic speciation system to definitively identify all gram-negative anaerobes. Definitive speciation of clostridia is useful in selected clinical settings. Definitive speciation of anaerobic cocci is usually not necessary except in research.

Limitations
1. Organisms isolated from inhibitory media may give false-negative and false-positive differentiation reactions.
2. The recommendations for therapy of the different groups are based on what is considered typical for each organism. Atypical resistance can occasionally occur with most organism groups. Therefore, therapy based on an organism's initial grouping must always be checked against actual *in vitro* results the following day.
3. Projection of which antibiotics are likely to be effective and ineffective are most likely to apply when the offending pathogen is the cause of a primary infection. They are less likely to apply if the pathogen is the cause of chronic or recurrent infection or if there are foreign objects or a structural abnormality at the site of infection. However, atypical resistance can occur at any infected site at any time.

9.2 BIOCHEMICAL IDENTIFICATION TESTS

9.2.1. Bacitracin Disk Susceptibility Test

Introduction
Taxo A disks are impregnated with a low level of bacitracin. It is used to differentiate Group A beta-hemolytic *Streptococcus* from other Lancefield

groups of hemolytic streptococci by the formation of a zone of inhibition around the disk.

Reagents and materials
Taxo A disk
5% Sheep blood agar plate
Sterile forceps

Procedure
1. Inoculate 5% sheep blood agar plate with the organism exhibiting beta-hemolysis.
2. With the use of sterile forceps, place a Taxo A disk onto inoculated plate.
3. Incubate plate in an atmosphere enriched with 5% to 10% CO_2 for 18 to 24 hours.
4. Observe plate for the presence of a zone of inhibition of streptococcal growth around the bacitracin disk.

Interpretation
Positive result = Zone of inhibition (Group A beta-hemolytic Streptococcus)
Negative result = No zone of inhibition (Group B–G beta-hemolytic streptococcus)
BBL Microbiology Systems, Cockeysville, Maryland.
Division of Becton Dickinson and Company, U.S.A.

9.2.2. Beta-Lactam Reagent Test

Introduction
Beta-lactam is a reagent disk containing a substrate (benzylpenicillin) and a pH indicator (bromcresol purple). This test is a quantitative, rapid acidometric method used to detect significant beta-lactamase–producing organisms, for instance, *Haemophilus influenzae, Neisseria gonorrhoeae,* and *Staphylococcus aureus.*

Reagents and materials
Reagent disk
Sterile water or saline at pH 6.5 to 7.2
Microscope slide
Applicator stick
Forceps

Procedure
1. Place a small drop of sterile water or saline at pH 6.5 to 7.2 on a microscopic slide.
2. With the use of sterile forceps, place the beta-lactam disk on the drop of diluent. Wait a few seconds for the disk to rehydrate.
3. Pick four to five well-isolated morphologically similar colonies from a young culture (18 to 24 hours) with a bacteriologic loop or wooden applicator stick.

4. Streak the colonies across the surface of the rehydrated disk.
5. Observe for color changes.

Interpretation
Positive result = Color changes from purple to yellow, indicating the production of beta-lactamase
Negative result = Disk remains purple, non–beta-lactamase

REFERENCE

Marion Scientific Reagents, Kansas City, Missouri 64114, Cat. #26-16-05.

9.2.3. Catalase Test

The organism to be tested should be grown on an agar slant heavily inoculated with a colony of the organism. The slant is usually incubated for 18 to 25 hours at optimal temperature. To test for catalase, set the slant in an inclined position and pour 1 mL 3% solution of hydrogen peroxide over the growth. The appearance of gas bubbles indicates a positive test.

An alternative to conducting the test with a slant culture is to emulsify a colony in 1 drop of 30% hydrogen peroxide (superoxol) on a glass slide. Immediate bubbling indicates a positive catalase test. Extreme care must be exercised if a colony is taken from a blood agar plate. The enzyme catalase is present in erythrocytes, and the carry-over of blood cells with the colony can give a false-positive reaction. Run controls with each batch of tests:

1. Positive control—*Staphylococcus aureus* ATCC strain
2. Negative control—*Streptococcus pyogenes* ATCC strain

9.2.4. Coagulase Test: Slide Method

Introduction
This test measures cell-associated coagulase or bound coagulase, which converts fibrinogen in plasma to fibrin, resulting in bacterial clumps. This is a characteristic of *Staphylococcus aureus*.

Reagents and materials
Staphylococcus species
Rabbit plasma (kept in the refrigerator or frozen in aliquots)
Normal saline solution

Procedure
1. Divide a microscopic slide into two sections.
2. Place 1 drop of normal saline on each section.
3. On each side, emulsify a colony of the suspected staphylococci.
4. Prepare in the same manner for positive and negative organisms.

5. Add 1 drop of undiluted rabbit plasma to each section.
6. Observe for white clumps or agglutination while mixing.

Interpretation
Positive result = *Staphylococcus aureus* (or *S. intermedius*)
Negative result = *Staphylococcus epidermidis* (or other species)

9.2.5. Coagulase Test Tube Method

Introduction
This test measures both cell-associated and cell-free coagulase. Cell-free coagulase cannot react directly with fibrinogen. It first must combine with a plasma factor (CRF = coagulase-reacting factor). Fibrinogen is converted to fibrin. This is a characteristic of *Staphylococcus aureus*.

Reagents and materials
Staphylococcus species
Rabbit plasma (kept in the refrigerator or frozen in aliquots)

Procedure
1. To 0.5 mL of 1:4 dilution of citrated plasma, add one loopful of growth from an 18- to 24-hour culture of *Staphylococcus*.
2. Incubate in a water bath or dry incubator at 37°C.
3. Examine for clotting at intervals of 30 minutes for 4 hours, again in 24 hours.

Interpretation
Positive result = *Staphylococcus aureus* or *S. intermedius*. Coagulase is represented by any degree of clotting from a loose clot suspended in plasma to a solid clot.
Negative result = *Staphylococcus epidermidis* and other species.

9.2.6. Germ Tube Test

Introduction
One of the most valuable tests for rapid presumptive identification of *Candida albicans* is the germ tube test. It is performed by mixing the suspected yeast cells with serum, then incubating for 2 to 4 hours at 37°C. The factors that may interfere with the formation of germ tubes are the following: using high concentration of yeast cells, temperature above 41°C or below 31°C, and heat-coagulated serum.

Reagents and materials
Human or sheep serum
Pasteur pipet
Microscopic slide
Test tube

Procedure

1. Using a Pasteur pipet, make a dilute suspension of the yeast colony in 0.5 to 1.0 mL human or sheep serum.
2. Incubate the mixture at 37°C for 2 to 4 hours.
3. Transfer a drop of suspension to a slide at the end of the 2 hours.
4. Examine the slide for hyphal elements or germ tubes at the end of 2 hours and, if negative, examine again after 4 hours.

Interpretation

Positive result = Germ tube without constrictions is about one-half the width and 3 to 4 times the length of the mother cell from which it develops. (*Candida albicans, Candida stellatoidea*)

Negative result = No germ tube formation (*Candida tropicalis*)

9.2.7. Indole Reagent Test

The reaction indicates the presence of the enzyme tryptophanase, which reacts with trytophane to produce indole. The indole produced reacts in the acid medium with the p-dimethylaminobenzaldehyde of indole reagent test to form a quinoidal red-violet compound.

Reagents and materials

Indole reagent droppers contain 0.5 mL 5% p-dimethyl-aminobenzaldehyde dissolved in a solution of 25% hydrochloric acid and 75% isobutyl alcohol. The reagent is hermetically sealed in a glass ampule, which affords protection of the solution from chemical instability until expiration date.

Procedure

1. To use indole reagent dropper, hold upright and point tip away from self. Grasp the middle with thumb and forefinger and squeeze gently to crush glass ampule inside the dropper.
2. Moisten a piece of Whatman No. 1 filter paper with a few drops of indole reagent.
3. Remove well-isolated colony to be tested with sterile loop or wooden stick. Then smear on moistened filter paper.
4. Observe the color change within 30 seconds.

Interpretation

Positive result = Red to purple color (*Escherichia coli*)

Negative result = Yellow to white color (*Klebsiella pneumoniae*)

REFERENCE

1. Marion Scientific Reagents, Kansas City, Missouri 64114, Cat. #26-11-81.

9.2.8. Mannitol Salt Agar Test

Introduction
Staphylococcus grows in media containing more than 7% salt concentration whereas other organisms cannot. Certain *Staphylococcus* species have enzymes that are capable of reducing sugar mannitol. When mannitol is reduced, there is an acid byproduct resulting in the pH color change of the agar.

Reagents and materials
Mannitol salt medium
Staphylococcus species
Wire loop

Procedure
1. Label one side of the mannitol salt as (+) control and the other side as (−) control.
2. To positive control, streak agar with *Staphylococcus aureus* and to negative control, streak agar with *Staphylococcus epidermidis*.
3. Into another mannitol salt agar, inoculate one to two colonies of suspected Staphylococcus.
4. Incubate both plates at 35°C in a non-CO_2 atmosphere for 18 to 24 hours.
5. Observe for color changes.

Interpretation
Positive result = Growth, yellow colonies of *Staphylococcus aureus*.
Negative result = Growth, pink colonies of *Staphylococcus epidermidis*.

NOTE: To confirm the particular species of Staphylococcus, all culture growth must be tested with other confirmatory tests such as coagulase, novobiocin, hemolysis, or Staph-Ident biochemical identification system (API).

9.2.9. Optochin Test

Introduction
Taxo P disks are impregnated with ethyl hydrocupreine hydrochloride (Optochin). It is used to differentiate *Streptococcus pneumoniae* from other alpha-hemolytic *Streptococcus* species by the formation of a zone of inhibition around Taxo P disks placed on a blood agar plate.

Reagents and materials
Taxo P disk
5% Sheep blood agar plate
Sterile forceps
Caliper

Procedure
1. Inoculate suspected organism onto 5% sheep blood agar plates.
2. With the use of sterile forceps, place a Taxo P disk onto inoculated plate.
3. Incubate plate aerobically at 35°C for 24 hours.
4. Measure the diameter of the zone obtained using a caliper.

Interpretation
Positive result = Zones of inhibition of 14 mm or more are formed with pure cultures of *Streptococcus pneumoniae*
Negative result = No zone of inhibition (Viridans *Streptococcus*)

REFERENCE

BBL Microbiology Systems. Division of Becton Dickinson and Company, U.S.A., Cockeysville, Maryland.

9.2.10. Oxidase Reagent Test

Introduction
The oxidase test is based on the bacterial production of an oxidase enzyme. This oxidase reaction is attributable to the cytochrome oxidase system, which activates in the presence of atmospheric oxygen, thereby oxidizing the phenylenediamine oxidase reagent to form a colored compound known as indophenol.

Reagents and materials
1. Cepti-Seal reagent droppers of oxidase reagent contain 0.5 mL 1% aqueous solution of N-tetramethyl-p-phenylenediamine dihydrochloride, which has been formulated with agents to insure maximum stability.
2. Whatman No. 1 Filter.

Procedure
1. Hold upright and point tip away from self. Grasp the middle with thumb and forefinger and squeeze gently to crush ampule inside the dropper. Tap bottom on table top a few times. Then invert for convenient drop-by-drop dispensing of the reagent.
2. Add a few drops of oxidase test reagent on a strip of filter paper. (Whatman No. 1 filter paper)
3. Streak a loopful of culture on the reagent-saturated paper with a platinum loop or applicator stick.
4. Observe the color change within 30 seconds.

Interpretation
Positive result = Violet to purple color (*Pseudomonas*, *Neisseria*)
Negative result = No change in color (*Escherichia coli*)

REFERENCE

Marion Scientific Reagents, Kansas City, Missouri 64114.

9.2.11. X and V Factor Strips

Introduction

Taxo strips impregnated with X, V, and XV factors are used in a qualitative procedure for the isolation and differentiation of *Haemophilus* species. The growth of these organisms is partially dependent on the presence of the X or V factor or both. These strips provide a simple method for determining the growth requirements of cultures in this group.

Reagents and materials

Taxo X and V Factor Strips, contain diphosphopyridine nucleotide (DPN)
Taxo X Factor Strips, contains Hemin
Taxo V Factor Strips, contains DPN
Mueller Hinton Agar
Forceps

Procedure

1. Inoculate suspected *Haemophilus* onto a Mueller Hinton Agar plate.
2. With the use of a sterile forceps, aseptically place Taxo X, V, and XV strips on the inoculated agar, leaving a distance of 20 mm between each strip.
3. Incubate at 35°C for 18 to 24 hours in a 5% to 10% CO_2 atmosphere.
4. Observe plate for growth around the strips.

Limitations: Because many X-Factor requiring organisms carry over X-Factor from the primary medium they may not be as reliable as commercially available ALA (8-aminolerulinic acid) impregnated paper disks from Remel Laboratories.

REFERENCE

BBL Microbiology Systems, Division of Becton Dickinson and Company, U.S.A., Cockeysville, Maryland.

Interpretation

Species	XV	V	X
H. influenzae	+	−	−
H. aegyptius	+	−	−
H. parainfluenzae	+	+	−
H. parahaemolyticus	+	+	−
H. haemolyticus	+	−	−
H. aphrophilus	+	+	+
H. paraphrophilus	+	+	−

9.2.12. Analytical Profile Index (API) Biochemical Identification

API 20 E Enterobacteriaceae

Introduction   The API 20 E System is a standardized, miniaturized version of conventional procedures for the identification of Enterobacteriaceae and other gram-negative bacteria. It is a ready-to-use microtube system designed for the performance of 23 standard biochemical tests from isolated colonies of bacteria on plating medium. Used in conjunction with the API Profile Recognition System, it is intended to assist laboratory personnel in identifying members of the family Enterobacteriaceae and other gram-negative bacteria accurately and easily. The API 20 E System has procedures for same-day and 18- to 24-hour identification of Enterobacteriaceae as well as 18- to 24- or 36- to 48-hour identification of other gram-negative bacteria. The biochemical identification of *Salmonella* (*S. arizonae*), Shigella, *E. coli* A through D, as well as *Vibrio choleras*, should be considered as presumptive identification and confirmed serologically.

Studies using cultures isolated from clinical specimens have established API 20 E as the most complete commercially available system for identification of Enterobacteriaceae. Clearcut reactions and ease of reading and interpretation permit valid comparison of results obtained each day in a particular laboratory, as well as valid comparison of results obtained in different laboratories worldwide.

Identification of Organisms   Identification of the organism can be made either with the aid of the differential charts or using the Profile Recognition System. When the differential charts are used to determine the identity of the cultures, the aggregate reactions given by the strains should be considered as a whole. Even when this is done, however, the conclusions reached may differ from laboratory to laboratory.

For rapid identification of species and biotype levels, the API Profile Recognition System Computer Service and Analytical Profile Indexes are available. A unique database compiled from strains of the collections of several institutions, as well as type and neotype cultures, allows precise statistical calculation and thus the identification of less commonly occurring microorganisms.

Quality Control   Biochemicals incorporated into the API 20 E System are quality controlled by standard testing procedures before their usage in the system. Each lot is controlled with stock cultures for sensitivity and specificity. In house quality control using stock cultures from the American Type Culture Collection (ATCC), Rockville, Maryland 20852, is recommended.

When lyophilized cultures are used for quality control procedures, several transfers should be made before the inoculation of 20 E. API recommends that the quality control be done using the 18- to 24-hour procedures. Same-day results for the recommended ATCC cultures are available from Technical Services, API.

Cultures
1. *Klebsiella pneumoniae* ATCC 13883
2. *Enterobacter cloacae* ATCC 13047
3. *Proteus vulgaris* ATCC 13315
4. *Pseudomonas aeruginosa* ATCC 10145

Interpretation

TUBE	POSITIVE	NEGATIVE
ONPG	Yellow	Colorless
ADH	Red or Orange	Yellow
LDC	Red or Orange	Yellow
ODC	Red or Orange	Yellow
CIT	Turquoise or Dark Blue	Light Green-Yellow
H$_2$S	Black Deposit	No deposit
URE	Red or Orange	Yellow
TDA	Add 1 Drop of 10%	Ferric Chloride
	Golden Brown to Red Brown	Yellow
IND	Add 1 Drop of	Kovacs Reagent
	Pink Red Ring	Yellow
VP	Add 1 drop of 40%	Potassium Hydroxide,
	then 1 drop of 6%	Alpha-Naphthol
	Pink-Red	Colorless
GEL	Diffusion or pigment	No diffusion
GLU	Yellow or Gray	Blue, Blue green or Green
	(at bottom or throughout tube)	
MAN		
INO	Yellow or Gray	Blue, Blue green,
SOR	(at the bottom of tube	or green
RHA	or throughout)	
SAC		
MEL		
AMY		
ARA		
GLU	After reading GLU reaction, add 2 drops of	
	0.8% sulfanilic acid and 2 drops 0.5% N,	
	N-dimethyl-alpha-naphthylamine	
Nitrate	NO$_2$ Red	Yellow
reduction	N$_2$ Gas Bubbles and	Orange after
AMY	yellow after	reagents[1] and
ARA	reagents[1] and	zinc
	zinc	

Add   NITRATE REDUCTION REACTION
                                   Glucose + or −
                             Observe for Gas Bubbles

Bubbles seen —— seen (Record Gas +)   No bubbles seen
      Add nitrate reagent   Add nitrate reagent
      Red   Yellow   Red   Yellow
   (Record NO$_2$ +) (Record NO$_2$ −)[2,3]   (Record NO$_2$+   (Record NO$_2$−)[2,3]
                                                        Gas)
                                                                    Add Zinc[3]
                                                                After 10 minutes
                                                   Pink-Orange Yellow
                                                   (Record Gas −)   (Record Gas +)

[1]2 drops 0.8% sulfanilic acid, 2 drops 0.5% N,N-dimethyl-alpha-naphthylamine.

[2]This reaction may be confirmed by the addition of zinc.

[3]Either zinc dust or 20-mesh granular zinc may be used. Zinc should be pushed to the bottom of the GLU cupula.

REFERENCE

API Analytab Products, Division of Sherwood Medical, New York.

API 20 A Anaerobe System

Introduction The API 20 A System allows rapid and reliable performance of 21 biochemical tests for routine species identification of anaerobes. Additional characteristics such as Gram reaction, colonial and microscopic morphology, and metabolic end products determined by gas–liquid chromatography should be considered in the identification of anaerobes.

Chemical and Physical Principles The API 20 A System consists of microtubes containing dehydrated substrates. These substrates are reconstituted by adding a bacterial suspension and incubated. The organisms react with the contents of the tubes and are read when the various indicator systems are affected by the metabolites or added reagents, after 24 hours' anaerobic incubation at 35° to 37°C.

Reagents and Materials
API 20 A System = strips, trays and lids, basal medium
Inoculating loop
Pasteur pipet
Mineral Oil
Phenol Red, 0.2%
H_2O_2* 3%

Procedure
1. *Preparation of Strips*
   a. Set up an incubation tray and lid.
   b. Dispense 5 mL tap water into the incubation tray (a plastic squeeze bottle may be used for this) to a humid atmosphere during incubation. This step can be eliminated if strips are incubated in an anaerobic jar.
   c. Remove the API strips from the sealed pouch and place one strip in each incubation tray.
2. *Preparation of Bacterial Suspension*
   Before inoculation of the API anaerobe basal medium, a pure culture of the anaerobic isolate must be obtained. To open the medium ampule, snap the top off by applying thumb pressure at the base of the flattened side of the plastic cap. Colonies should be picked from a fresh culture on a nonselective medium, using a swab or loop. Hold the tube in a slanted position and emulsify the colonies in the medium as quickly as possible by sliding the swab or loop along the side of the vial to minimize aeration. Replace the plastic cap. The final density of the suspension should be equal to or greater than that of a No. 3 McFarland.
3. *Inoculation of the Strips*
   The API 20 A strips contain 20 microtubes, each of which consists of a tube and a cupula section.

The microtubes are inoculated under aerobic conditions and then placed in an anaerobic system for incubation, unless an anaerobic chamber is used, which allows inoculation and incubation under anaerobic conditions.

a. Remove the cap from the ampule containing inoculum. Insert and fill a sterile, 5-mL Pasteur pipet.

b. Tilt the incubation tray and fill the tube section of the microtubes by placing the pipet tip against the side of the cupula.

c. After inoculation, completely fill the cupula of the GEL tube.

d. After inoculation, completely fill the cupula section of the IND tube with sterile mineral oil.

After inoculation of the API 20 A strip, the same bacterial suspension can be used for inoculating other differential media, egg yolk agar, medium for GLC analysis, or a holding medium such as chopped meat glucose broth. As a final step, plate out a sample from the medium inoculum to check the viability of the culture. After use, the ampule should be autoclaved, incinerated, or immersed in a germicide before disposal.

4. *Methods of Incubation by Ano 2 Jar Technique*

GasPak anaerobic jars should be used in a horizontal position to incubate the API 20 A strips. After inoculation of the API 20 A strip, remove it from the incubation tray and place it in the API 20 A Holder. After all the strips have been inoculated or the strip holder is filled, cut and place the GasPak generator envelope in the center of the holder in a horizontal position. Add water to the envelope, then slide the holder into the Ano 2 jar. Include a methylene blue chemical strip indicator to check anaerobiosis. Place the lid containing activated catalyst on the jar lid and incubate the strips for 24 hours at 35° to 37°C.

5. *Reading the Strips*

After 24 hours' incubation, the strips are removed from anaerobic conditions and the interpretation of reactions is performed.

a. One drop of Bromcresol purple should be added to ALL microtubes containing carbohydrates.

b. Add 2 drops xylene to the mineral oil overlay on indo (IND) microtube: mix well (in cupula) with applicator stick and wait 2 to 3 minutes, add 1 drop of Ehrlich's reagent.

c. Catalase production is determined after strips have been exposed to air for 30 minutes. Add 2 drops 3% H_2O_2 to the microtube containing mannitol (MAN).

d. After all reactions have been recorded on the report sheet and satisfactory identification has been made, the API 20 A strip or incubation tray must be autoclaved, incinerated, or immersed in a germicide before disposal.

Identification of Organisms   Identification of organisms can be made with the aid of the differential charts or by using the Analytical Profile Index. When differential charts are used to determine the identity of cultures, the aggregate reactions given by the strains should be considered as a whole. Even when this is done, however, the conclusions reached may differ from laboratory to laboratory. The nomenclature used is that of Virginia Polytechnic Institute.

Quality Control   Biochemicals incorporated into the API 20 A system are quality controlled by standard testing procedures before their usage in the system. Each lot is controlled with stock cultures for sensitivity and specificity. For those who wish to do their own quality control testing, the use of stock cultures from the American Type Culture Collection, Rockville, Maryland 20852, is recommended.

CULTURES:
1. *Clostridium histolyticum*   ATCC 19401
2. *Bacteroides ovatus*   ATCC 8483
3. *Propionibacterium acnes*   ATCC 11827
4. *Clostridium sordellii*   ATCC 9714
5. *Clostridium perfringens*   ATCC 13124

API Analytab Products, Division of Sherwood Medical, New York.

API 20 C Clinical Yeast System

Introduction   API 20 C is a ready-to-use micromethod that permits the performance of 1% assimilation tests for the identification of most clinically significant yeasts and yeastlike organisms. Biochemical reactions are complete after 72 hours' incubation at 30°C.

Chemical and physical principles   The API 20 C System consists of a series of cupula containing dehydrated substrates. These substrates are reconstituted by the addition of a pure yeast suspension in API 20 C Basal Medium to the cupulas. The strips are incubated at 30°C and read at 24-, 48-, and 72-hour intervals.

Reagents and materials
API 20 C System = strips, trays and lids, basal medium
Inoculating loop
Pasteur pipets
Water
Boiling chips
Sabouraud's dextrose agar plates

Procedure
1. *Preparation of strips*
   a. Set up an incubation tray and lid.
   b. Record the patient's specimen number on the elongated flap of the tray.
   c. Dispense 10 mL water into the incubation tray to provide a humid atmosphere during incubation. A plastic squeeze bottle may be used for this.
   d. Remove the API strip from the sealed envelope and place on strip in each incubation tray.
2. *Preparation of yeast suspension*
   a. Allow the ampules of basal medium to come to room temperature before use.

Interpretation

TUBE	POSITIVE	NEGATIVE
IND	*Add two drops xylene to oil. Add 1 drop Ehrlich's Reagent.	Yellow
URE	Red	Yellow or orange
GLU, MAN, LAC, SAC	Yellow or	Purple
HAL, SAL, XYL, ARA	Yellow Red	
GLY, CEL, MNE, MLZ		
RAF, SOR, RHA, TRE		
GEL	Liquefaction of Black particles	No liquefaction of black particles
ESC	Negative fluorescence	Positive fluorescence
CAT	Add 2 drops 3% H_2O_2—bubbles	No bubbles

   b. Place the ampules in a container with boiling chips and a sufficient quantity of water to float the ampules. Cover container. Bring to boil. Allow the ampules to remain in the boiling water for 5 minutes after the medium appears melted to assure complete liquefication.
   c. Place the container with the boiled ampules directly into a water bath set at 50°C +2°C and allow the ampules to cool for 10 to 20 minutes.
   d. To open the medium ampule, snap the top off by applying thumb pressure at the base of the flattened side of the plastic cap.
   e. From a fresh culture of 48 to 72 hours' growth on Sabouraud's dextrose agar, prepare a yeast suspension in the API 20 C basal medium.
3. *Inoculation of the Strips*
    The API 20 C strip contains 20 ampules. With a sterile pipet, inoculate each cupula by placing the pipet tip against the side of the cupula, avoiding bubble formation. Completely fill the cupula with the yeast suspension. The suspension in all cupula should be slightly convex. After use the ampule must be disposed of in a biohazard container or autoclaved before disposal.
4. *Incubation of the Strips*
    After inoculation, place the lid on the tray and incubate for 72 hours at 27° to 30°C. A beaker of water may be placed inside the incubator in increase humidity.
5. *Reading the Strips*
    a. Read reactions at 24, 48, and 72 hours of incubation period at 27° to 30°C and record on worksheet or indicate in computer.
    b. The cupula with "O" serves as a negative control for assimilation reactions. Cupulas showing turbidity significantly heavier than the O cupula are positive.
    c. After reading and interpreting all reactions and recording these on worksheet or in computer and satisfactory identification has been made, the entire tray must be autoclaved before disposal.

Identification of Organism   Identification of organisms can be made with the aid of differential charts included with the API 20 C Analytical Profile Index.

Consider the aggregate reactions as a whole when using differential charts. It may be advantageous to submit rare yeast isolates and their profiles to the research mycology laboratory or reference laboratory for confirmation and further study.

Quality Control   Biochemicals incorporated into the API 20 C system are quality controlled by standard testing procedures before their use in the system. However, it is recommended that laboratories do their own quality control using the ATCC stock cultures, with which known reactions are obtained. This is usually performed which each lot number or package opened and may be set up as monthly quality control procedure if desired.

Interpretation
Positive—Growth significantly greater than "O" control and generally comparable to GLU cupula.
Negative—No growth or growth comparable to that of the "O" control.

Limitations   If the inoculum is too heavy, "carry-over" in some cupulas may interfere with the interpretation. A halo in the lower portion of the INO cupula may be present and should not be interpreted as a positive reaction.

REFERENCE

API Analytab Products, New York.
Package Insert, API Analytab Products, New York.

API 20 S Streptococcus System
The API 20 S System is similar to the Staph-Ident system in procedure. The conventional and chromogenic tests for the identification of streptococci and aerococci are based on the biochemical tests proposed by Facklam for streptococcal groups A,B, enterococcal D, non-enterococcal D, and viridans. The API 20 S system, when used alone or in conjunction with the analytical profile index, enables laboratorians to identify *Streptococcus pyogenes, S. agalactiae, S. pneumoniae, S. avium, S. faecium,* and others (primarily Lancefield Groups A, B, and beta-hemoloytic streptococci groups C, F, or G and group D to the species level) and *Aerococcus.*

Procedure   The preparation of microcupula for inoculation and incubation is done according to the same protocol as "Staph-Ident" procedure described previously subject to the following variations:

Incubation period is shortened to only 4 hours
Reagents employed: Ninhydrin and Cinnamaldehyde reagent

Reading of Strips

1. After 4 hours' incubation, record the results for all tests not requiring reagents (i.e., BEM through ARG). Reaction interpretation can be found in the summary of results.

2. Add 1 drop Cinnamaldehyde reagent to microcupulas LEU, SER, PYR, and ARL. Record any reactions that occur within 1 minute. Disregard any reaction occurring after 1 minute.
3. Perform the HIP test:
   a. Add 4 drops Ninhydrin reagent to HIP microcupula.
   b. A positive result is indicated if a dark blue color develops immediately.
   c. Place all other strips in incubator at 35° to 37°C and leave for 5 to 10 minutes. After incubation, record HIP reaction per summary interpretation.
4. After recording all reactions and a satisfactory identification has been made, entire incubation unit must be autoclaved before disposal.

Identification of Streptococci   Identification of the various species of streptococci can be made using the API 20 S Streptococcus Analytical Profile Index or with the aid of the package insert differential chart.

Quality Control   Tests incorporated into the API 20 S System are quality controlled before use. However, each lot should be controlled by in-use testing using stock ATCC cultures, Rockville, Maryland. Recommended cultures should include:

Streptococcus pyogenes
Streptococcus agalactiae
Streptococcus faecalis
Streptococcus durans
Streptococcus bovis
Streptococcus avium

Interpretation   See manufacturer's package insert for specifics. Generally, positive reactions for BEM are black and negative is a tan to light gray. MAN-to SBS-positive results are indicated by yellow or yellow-orange reactions, with a negative varying from colorless to red or red-orange. INA is positive if a blue or dark blue color develops and negative if clear or very light blue. RAF to TRE are positive if yellow or yellow-orange and negative if not. For LEU to ARL after addition of Cinnamaldehyde, a pink or purple indicates a positive result and yellow or light orange color is considered negative. Hemolysis is incorporated into the identification scheme as seen on blood agar and recorded as beta for positive and alpha (green or partial hemolysis) or gamma (no hemolysis) is recorded as negative.

Substrate	Positive	Negative
PHS	Yellow	Clear or straw-colored
URE	Purple to red-orange	Yellow or orange-yellow
GLS	Yellow	Clear or straw-colored
MNE	Yellow or yellow-orange	Red or orange
MAN	Yellow or yellow-orange	Red or orange
TRE	Yellow or yellow-orange	Red or orange
SAL	Yellow or yellow-orange	Red or orange

GLC	Yellow	Clear or straw-colored
ARG	Purple to red-orange	Yellow or yellow-orange
After addition of reagent:		
NGP	Plum-purple	Yellow or colorless

REFERENCE

API Analytab, New York, U.S.A.

BIBLIOGRAPHY

Balows A (Ed.): Manual of clinical microbiology, 5th Edition. Washington, DC: American Society for Microbiology, 1991.

Baron EJ, Peterson L, Finegold SM (Eds.): Bailey and Scott's diagnostic microbiology, 9th Edition. St. Louis: C.V. Mosby, 1994.

Koneman EW: Color atlas and textbook of diagnostic microbiology, 4th Edition. Philadelphia: J.B. Lippincott, 1992.

Wegner DL: Session 47, 1993 Northwest Symposium by the Pacific Area Resource Office of the National Laboratory Training Network and Centers for Disease Control, 1993.

Wegner DL, Schrantz RD: Rapid, inexpensive identification of commonly encountered aerobic gram negative bacilli. Lab Med 1984;15:52–54.

Polymerase Chain Reaction

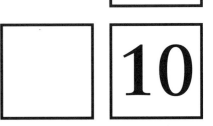

Polymerase chain reaction (PCR) was first described in 1985 and is an extremely sensitive method designed to amplify and detect selected target DNA sequences (Saiki et al. 1985). The technique has been used primarily in research and clinical studies of genetic disorders, infectious diseases, forensic medicine, and oncology. PCR is based on the principle that a target DNA sequence (usually one hundred to several hundred base pairs) can be synthesized *in vitro* by the enzyme DNA polymerase. Repeated cycles of synthesis result in amplification of the DNA sequence, which then can be detected.

Samples to be tested by PCR for the presence of infectious agents can be frozen because only DNA, and not viable organisms, is required. A temperature of −20°C is acceptable for freezing, but −70°C or −80°C is preferable, especially for longer-term storage. In preparation for the PCR procedure, whole genomic DNA must be extracted from the sample (fresh or frozen) to be tested. There are several means to accomplish this. In general, fluids such as cerebrospinal fluid and aqueous or vitreous humor can be heated at 95°C for 30 minutes. Samples such as blood or tissues that contain cells are treated with a proteinase K (final concentration, 250 μg/mL)/detergent solution for 1 hour at 56°C and then heat denatured at 95°C for 10 minutes. The detergent solubilizes the cell components and the proteinase K digests the proteins. Commercially available products such as GeneReleaser (BioVentures Inc., Murfreezboro, Tennessee) can also be used to release genomic DNA. Alternatively, DNA may be purified from samples to be tested by PCR by using a phenol/chloroform extraction procedure. Methods for extraction of DNA from formalin-fixed or paraffin-embedded tissues have also been reported (Rogers et al. 1990).

142

General procedures for PCR amplifications are available in several recent publications and reviews (Sambrook et al. 1989; Innis et al. 1990; Erlich et al. 1991). Specific procedures can be obtained from the literature for the target DNA of interest. Amplifications are performed in a small volume, usually 100 μL or less. A PCR reaction mix is prepared that contains (1) 10× amplification buffer; standard buffer contains 0.5 mol/L potassium chloride, 10 mmol/L Tris HCl (pH 8.3), 15 mmol/L magnesium chloride, and 0.1% gelatin. The free magnesium concentration is critical for functioning of the DNA polymerase and should be optimized for each primer/target system. (2) DNA polymerase from the bacterium *Thermus acquaticus* (Taq polymerase) survives the repeated high-temperature denaturations in the PCR procedure and is used at a concentration of approximately 2 units, which is depleted after approximately 30 amplification cycles. (3) Equimolar concentrations of all four deoxynucleotide triphosphates (dNTPs: dATP, dCTP, dGTP, and dTTP),* 200 μmol/L each. (4) Oligonucleotide primers: 1 μmol/L is usually sufficient for approximately thirty amplification cycles. For target DNA to be amplified by PCR, the nucleotide sequences at either end of the DNA piece must be known. Primers are short pieces of single-stranded DNA (preferably twenty to twenty-four nucleotides in length) that are complementary to these known sequences. Primers should ideally have a guanine plus cytosine content of approximately 50%, should not contain guanine–cytosine-rich stretches, and should not contain any homologous regions between the oligonucleotides that constitute the primer pair. Primers can be made synthetically and are designed to anneal to the end regions of the target DNA to serve as an initiation point for synthesis. (5) The sample to be tested. (6) Sterile distilled water to bring the volume to 100 μL. Once the water, buffer, deoxyribonucleoside triphosphates (dNTPs), primer pairs, polymerase, and sample are combined in a microcentrifuge tube, the mixture is microcentrifuged to consolidate the reagents and is overlaid with 100 μL mineral oil to prevent evaporation of the mixture during amplification. A positive control and a negative buffer control are included with each reaction. It is also suggested that a conserved sequence (such as human leukocyte antigen DQR or hypoxanthine-guanine phosphoribosyl transferase [HPRT]) present in the genome of all human cells concurrently be amplified from the test sample to confirm the integrity of the DNA and to demonstrate that no inhibitors of the Taq polymerase are present.

The amplification reaction is driven entirely by a succession of temperature changes and is usually carried out in an automated thermocycler. The specific temperatures used for a given amplification reaction need to be optimized for that particular reaction. For DNA synthesis to begin, a single-stranded DNA template is required, along which the Taq polymerase can place new oligonucleotides. Most DNA samples to be analyzed are double stranded. The amplification process, therefore, starts with denaturation of double-stranded DNA

*(dNTP = deoxynucleotide triphosphate,
 dATP = 2'-deoxyadenosine 5'-triphosphate,
 dCTP = 2'-deoxycytidine 5'-triphosphate,
 dGTP = 2'deoxyguanosine 5'-triphosphate,
 dTTP = 2'-deoxythymidine 5'-triphosphate)

into two single strands. This is done at higher temperatures (94° to 96°C). In the next step, the oligonucleotide primers are annealed to the appropriate sites on the target single-stranded DNA at a lower temperature (25° to 60°C). Enzymatic DNA synthesis occurs at 72°C and consists of extension of the primer by inserting the appropriate dNTPs, using the target DNA as a template. Extension occurs along both strands of DNA and occurs from each primer toward the other. The timing of each step needs to be optimized, depending on the length of the DNA sequence to be amplified. The result is that where there was initially a single copy of the target DNA sequence, now there are two. The new DNA pieces then can serve also as templates in subsequent rounds of denaturation, annealing, and DNA synthesis. With each cycle, the amount of target DNA is doubled and approximately 25 to 30 cycles can produce a 10^5- to 10^6-fold increase in the target sequence. If additional amplification is needed, the amplified DNA can be diluted and reamplified an additional 25 to 30 cycles in a new PCR reaction. This procedure results in a final 10^9- to 10^{10}-fold increase in the target sequence.

Amplified DNA is generally separated and visualized using ethidium bromide/agarose gel electrophoresis. DNA-grade ultrapure agarose, polyacrylamide, or high-density (NuSieve, InterMountain Scientific, Bountiful, Utah) gels can be used. Ethidium bromide can be added during preparation of the gel and is used at a final concentration of 0.5 µg/mL or the gel may be stained after electrophoresis. The samples are mixed with a $10\times$ loading buffer containing glycerol and bromophenol blue and loaded into the wells of the gel. Molecular weight markers are also mixed with loading buffer and run in parallel with the samples.

Electrophoresis is done in Tris-Borate/ethylenediaminetetra-acetic acid (EDTA) buffer until the bromophenol blue dye approaches the bottom of the gel. The amplified DNA fragments then are visualized using a long-wave ultraviolet light (see Figure 10.1). The sizes of the amplified bands are determined by comparing their locations relative to the molecular weight marker panel. The expected size of the amplified fragment of the positive control is predetermined from the known DNA sequence. Test samples demonstrating positive bands of the same molecular weight as the control are considered to be positive. The identity of the amplified product may be further confirmed by a method such as dot blot, slot blot, or Southern blot hybridization with a ^{32}P–end-labeled probe. Other postamplification detection formats have been reported and are being evaluated.

Because of the extreme sensitivity of the system, it is essential to avoid false-positives, which could occur by cross-contamination between samples or by contamination of reagents with amplified products or positive controls. Some general precautions to minimize the risk of contamination include performing the initial processing in a biologic safety hood not used for any other PCR-related procedures. All reagents should be prepared in another biologic safety cabinet, using materials dedicated solely to PCR, and should be aliquoted into sterile tubes before use. Amplified products and procedures for their detection and confirmation should be separated from the other reagents and are preferably handled in another laboratory. In addition to the general precautions mentioned, a modification of PCR has been developed that enzymatically destroys any DNA that has been carried over from previous amplifications (Longo et al.

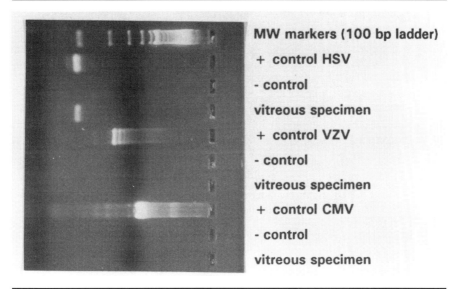

Figure 10.1
10-μL aliquots of amplified product with 1-μL loading buffer were run on a 3:1
NuSieve agarose gel stained with ethidium bromide. Lane 1 contains molecular weight
standards ranging from 10 to 1000 base pairs in increments of 100. Lane 2 shows a
specific band of 92 base pairs, which represents a positive reaction for herpes simplex
virus in a control culture of HSV-infected cells. Lane 5 shows a positive band at 224
base pairs for a control specimen of VZV, and lane 8 shows a CMV positive band at
435 base pairs. Lanes 3, 6, and 9 are negative controls (PCR reaction mixture with all
reagents except DNA) for their respective reactions. Lane 4 shows an amplified vitreous biopsy specimen from a patient with acute retinal necrosis that is positive for
HSV. Lanes 7 and 10 show the same vitreous specimen to be negative for both VZV
and CMV.

1990). In this modification, deoxyuridine triphosphate is substituted for de-
oxythymidine triphosphate and is incorporated into the amplification product.
In this way, amplified PCR products can be distinguished from natural sample
DNA. The enzyme uracil-DNA-glycosylase is added to the starting reaction
mixture in subsequent reactions. The enzyme is activated by heating the mixture to 56°C, allowed to react for 10 minutes, and then denatured by heating
at 94°C for 10 minutes. The uracil-DNA-glycosylase excises uracil from any
carry over DNA present in the reaction and eliminates it before the first cycle
of standard amplification begins.

Several modifications of the standard PCR procedure have been introduced
in attempt to increase the sensitivity and specificity of the system. To minimize
amplification of nontarget DNA sequences, some investigators have employed
a "hot start" system in which the DNA polymerase, magnesium chloride, and
primers are added to the reaction mixture only after it has reached a temperature of greater than 70°C (Faloona et al. 1990). Another system sometimes used
to increase specificity involves the use of "nested primers" (Mullis and Faloona

1987). In this system, the initial PCR amplification is followed by additional amplification using primers specific for a target sequence that is internal to the primers previously used. The product of the second amplification is then a subset of the original target sequence.

Sequences of RNA also can be used as a template for PCR in a procedure called "reverse transcriptase PCR" (Saiki et al. 1988, Noonan and Robinson 1988). The mRNA must first be converted to a cDNA intermediate by the enzyme reverse transcriptase. The cDNA then can be used as a template in conventional PCR. Amplification of mRNA can be useful; detection of a specific mRNA gives an indication of active gene expression rather than indicating only the presence of a specific DNA sequence.

New applications for PCR are continuously being developed, and PCR has found a place in both clinical and research medicine. Before being implemented for routine diagnostic purposes, the sensitivities and specifications of PCR need to be determined and standardized. Preliminary experimental data show the technique to have great promise, especially when only small-sized samples can be obtained, as is often the case with ocular specimens. Also, the diagnosis of infectious diseases with atypical presentations, as occurs often in immune-compromised patients, may be facilitated by PCR. Because PCR requires only DNA and does not require living tissue or pathogens, the technique may be useful in the evaluation of specimens obtained in field studies, where it may be difficult to maintain viability.

The ophthalmic literature has a rapidly growing number of publications in which PCR is used. Most of these studies have a research orientation, although clinical diagnostic applications are becoming more prominent. An attempt has not been made here to give an exhaustive review of the literature; however, the following summaries are presented as examples of some of the uses of PCR in ophthalmology.

Herpes simplex virus (HSV)

The diagnosis of active HSV corneal disease is based primarily on clinical appearance. In cases presenting as typical dendritic keratitis, the diagnosis is usually straightforward, and virologic diagnostic tests are not routinely performed. However, recent descriptions of varicella-zoster virus (VZV) and Epstein-Barr virus (EBV) infections of the cornea indicate that these viruses also may be associated with dendrites and should be considered in the differential diagnosis of dendritic keratitis. Rapid culture techniques, which give results within 24 hours, are available for detection of HSV in clinical specimens. Even when HSV cultures have been performed on ocular specimens under ideal conditions, however, isolation rates have been variable, and it has been suggested that this may be because of the presence of only low levels of virus in the cornea even during active infection. PCR may be advantageous in these cases because very low levels of virus can be detected using PCR, and results are available within several hours. PCR also may be helpful for patients presenting with stromal HSV disease, in which the clinical diagnosis may be more difficult because other infections such as *Acanthamoeba* may present similarly.

Several research studies have used PCR to add to our understanding of the mechanisms underlying herpetic keratitis and the mechanisms of latency of

HSV in the cornea. One such study used PCR to investigate whether the cornea is a site for HSV latency in previously actively infected eyes (Rong et al. 1991). DNA was extracted from eighteen corneal buttons from patients undergoing keratoplasty who had an original diagnosis of HSV based on clinical appearance and positive cultures. These samples were compared with the DNA extracted from corneal buttons from other transplant patients who did not carry a diagnosis of HSV, as well as with buttons from cadaveric donor eyes. Primer pairs were chosen to detect the latency-associated transcript (LAT) gene and thymidine kinase (TK) gene, both of which are associated with latency. Positive results were obtained in 94% of the previously infected cornea samples, and most of these were found to contain both the LAT and TK genes. Control corneas were all negative. These findings lead to the conclusion that HSV can establish latency in the cornea and can be detected by PCR in quiescent tissue.

Another study that addressed the question of HSV latency in the cornea used PCR to investigate the pattern of HSV gene expression in corneal buttons obtained at transplantation (Kaye et al. 1991). Ten patients with a history of HSV keratitis were evaluated, as were ten patients with corneal disease not involving HSV and three cadaveric donor corneas. All but one of the cadaver donors had serum antibodies to HSV, indicating prior exposure to the virus. Standard PCR was used to identify DNA sequences from the TK, glycoprotein C (GC), and major capsid protein (MCP) genes. All three HSV genes were detected in each of ten patients with a history of HSV keratitis and in five of the ten patients with corneal disease not caused by HSV. The three donor controls were negative. Reverse transcriptase PCR, which is used to detect mRNA, showed that viral gene transcription was limited to the LAT gene in eight of eight patients with prior HSV keratitis and in three of the five positive patients in the diseased cornea not caused by HSV group. This study concluded that the whole HSV genome is present but can be maintained in latent state not always associated with disease.

Cytomegalovirus (CMV)

Because CMV typically grows slowly in culture and is treated with ganciclovir or foscarnet rather than acyclovir, which is used to treat HSV and VZV, a rapid means of establishing a diagnosis is important. PCR has been shown to be useful for identification of CMV in aqueous, vitreous, and subretinal fluid specimens from patients with acquired immune deficiency syndrome (AIDS) and clinical CMV retinitis (Fox et al. 1991). All patients were undergoing treatment with intravenous ganciclovir. Specimens were obtained during vitrectomy for retinal detachment and were compared with aqueous and vitreous specimens from normal human immunodeficiency virus (HIV)-negative patients undergoing routine cataract extraction or vitrectomy for retinal disease other than retinitis. CMV DNA was amplified from nine of nine vitreous specimens, five of five subretinal fluid specimens, and three of three aqueous specimens from patients with retinitis. Two of two vitreous specimens and two of two aqueous specimens obtained at autopsy from AIDS patients with retinitis were also positive for CMV DNA. One patient with AIDS but no retinitis also had CMV DNA identifiable in vitreous, as did one control patient without AIDS or retinitis. All control aqueous specimens were negative. All specimens were tested also for the presence of HSV and EBV DNA by PCR and were negative in each case.

Another study used ocular specimens from sixteen patients with AIDS. The specimens were obtained at autopsy and paraffin embedded or formalin fixed (Biswas et al. 1993). They then were evaluated by light microscopy, *in situ* hybridization, and PCR. For PCR, two primer sets were used, one to detect the immediate early antigen and one to detect the late antigen (gp64) of CMV. CMV DNA was detected by PCR in six specimens. Both primers were positive in two of the six cases, and the late antigen primers detected CMV in the remaining four positive specimens. Four of the PCR-positives also were found to be positive by *in situ* hybridization using biotin-labeled probes. This study showed PCR to be more sensitive than *in situ* DNA hybridization and points out the importance of selection of appropriate primers.

Epstein-Barr virus (EBV)
Epstein-Barr virus infections of the cornea present as dendritic or stromal keratitis that can resemble the corneal infection caused by HSV. Diagnosis by isolation of the virus in culture requires human umbilical cord blood mononuclear cells and is generally not available. PCR may be a particularly useful technique for the detection of EBV and has been applied to a variety of ocular specimens, including cornea, aqueous, and vitreous (Fox et al. 1991, Crouse et al. 1990). One case report used PCR to aid in the diagnosis of a recurrent dendritic keratitis in a patient who had received a chemical facial peeling treatment (Pflugfelder et al. 1990a). When cultures for HSV and VZV were negative, corneal epithelial scrapings were tested by PCR with primers to detect the *Bam*HI K gene of EBV, followed by Southern blot hybridization. EBV DNA was detected by PCR in this specimen and it was believed that EBV was reactivated from latently infected cells by phorbol esters in the croton oil peeling solution.

Another study was done using PCR to evaluate the role of EBV in the pathogenesis of Sjögren's syndrome, which often occurs after an acute EBV infection (Pflugfelder et al. 1990b). Using primers to detect the *Bam*HI K gene of EBV and Southern blot hybridization for confirmation of identity of amplified product, EBV DNA sequences were detected in five of ten (50%) peripheral blood mononuclear preparations and in eight of ten (80%) lacrimal gland and tear film specimens from patients with Sjögren's syndrome. This recovery rate was found to be statistically significantly greater when compared with that for specimens obtained from EBV-seropositive individuals without Sjögren's syndrome, in which 11 of 34 (32%) of lacrimal glands were positive for EBV but all peripheral blood mononuclear cell and tear specimens were negative.

Human immunodeficiency virus (HIV-1) / human herpesvirus-6 (HHV-6)
PCR has been used to detect HIV-1 DNA in high-risk individuals before they develop a serologic response (Loch and Mach 1988) and in patients who are seropositive but culture negative (Ou et al. 1988). The technique also has been useful in detection of active infection in antibody-positive neonates, where there may be a question of true infection versus presence of passive maternal

antibody (Rogers et al. 1989). PCR has also been used to evaluate sections of corneal buttons obtained at autopsy for the presence of HIV-1 and HHV-6 in HIV-positive patients (Qavi et al. 1991). Thirty-five pairs of corneal buttons (70 eyes) were obtained from asymptomatic HIV-positive patients and were compared to 10 pair of corneas (20 eyes) from symptomatic patients with AIDS and four corneas from normal HIV-negative patients. Three of the 70 corneas from asymptomatic HIV-positive patients were found to harbor both HIV-1 and HHV-6. Also, three of the 20 corneas from AIDS patients were found to contain both HIV-1 and HHV-6. All six corneas that were positive by PCR were also positive for HIV-1 by culture. None of the four control corneas had HIV-1 or HHV-6 detectable by PCR. This study confirmed that HIV-1 and HHV-6 can invade human corneal tissues. The significance of the presence of either of these viruses in the cornea is not known.

Herpesvirus panel

The studies presented above indicate that PCR can be successfully used to identify infections caused by members of the herpesvirus group in ocular tissues. There are circumstances (i.e., immunocompromised patients with rapidly progressing retinal necrosis) where evaluation of specimens using a panel of primers to detect each of the herpesviruses may be beneficial. One preliminary study evaluated vitreous biopsy samples from 40 patients with clinically diagnosed viral retinitis and compared them to 40 control patients without retinal disease (Mitchell et al. 1993). A panel of PCR primers to detect HSV-1, HSV-2, VZV, CMV, VZV, EBV, and HHV-6 in a nested PCR system was used. VZV and CMV were found in significantly more patients with retinitis than in the control group. No significant difference between the two groups was found with HSV-1, HSV-2, EBV, or HHV-6.

One study used a similar panel of primers to evaluate corneal epithelium from cadaveric donor eyes (Crouse et al. 1990). Thirty-four samples of corneal epithelium and nine samples of conjunctival epithelium were obtained from 22 donor eyes. These were compared with samples of corneal epithelium from eight patients with clinically diagnosed epithelial or dendritic keratitis. The PCR primers were chosen to detect CMV (gp 64 gene), EBV (Bam HI K) gene, and HSV (ICPO region). EBV DNA was detected in 3 donor corneal epithelium specimens and HSV in one. EBV was also detected in one case of atypical peripheral dendritic keratitis. Three of the remaining seven diseased cornea controls were positive for HSV by PCR and by routine culture. This study indicates that herpesviruses can be detected in a small percentage of normal donor corneas, suggesting, because of the potential for transmission via transplantation, that PCR be used to screen Eye Bank donor eyes.

Human papillomavirus (HPV)

PCR has been used to identify HPV DNA in several studies of conjunctival and corneal dysplasias and carcinomas. Lauer et al. (1990) used PCR to detect HPV DNA in five biopsy specimens from patients with conjunctival intraepithelial neoplasia. Primers were designed to detect the E6 ORF region of the genome associated with the potential for malignant transformation of type 16 and type

18 HPV. Radiolabeled probes were used to confirm the amplified product. Results showed the presence of HPV type 18 in two specimens and HPV type 16 in four specimens, including two specimens that contained both types of HPV.

Another study used PCR with primers to detect the E1 consensus segment of HPV followed by Southern blot hybridization to investigate three cases of conjunctival squamous cell dysplasias presenting bilaterally in various stages of the disease (Odrich et al. 1991). HPV DNA was detected in all specimens, indicating that HPV can be associated with a variety of conjunctival abnormalities ranging from inflammatory lesions and dysplasias to invasive carcinoma. Based on these findings and the risk of milder lesions eventually culminating in carcinoma, the authors recommended that all conjunctival lesions with a diffuse, hypertrophic, or hyperkeratotic appearance be biopsied and analyzed by PCR.

A larger series used PCR to examine 42 paraffin-embedded specimens from 38 patients with conjunctival lesions ranging from mild dysplasia to invasive carcinoma (McDonnell et al. 1992). The primers used were the same as those used by Lauer et al., described above, to detect HPV 16 and 18, and amplified products were confirmed by dot blot hybridization. DNA from HPV 16 was detected in 37 of the 38 specimens. HPV type 18 was not detected in any of the specimens. In this study, four patients who had two separate surgeries had HPV DNA in specimens from both surgeries. Also in ten patients there were multiple specimens from the same surgery and all of the specimens were positive. Interestingly, HPV DNA was also present in four of six swab specimens taken from limbal tissue in the contralateral eyes of patients with unilateral involvement. HPV DNA was also detected in both the involved and uninvolved eye in one patient eight years after successful surgical excision of the lesion in the involved eye. It was concluded that the presence of HPV does not indicate a hyperplastic process and that some other factor, possibly ultraviolet light exposure, must be present.

Chlamydia

Chlamydia infections have been relatively extensively studied using PCR. Urethral and endocervical specimens subjected to PCR in several studies have shown that PCR is at least as sensitive as *Chlamydia* culture and has the advantage of being more rapid. Conjunctival specimens from patients with follicular conjunctivitis have also been evaluated by PCR (Talley et al. 1992). Primers specific for the major outer membrane protein (MOMP) of *C. trachomatis* were used in a uracil-N-glycosylase PCR system. Using this system, four of 30 specimens were positive. Three of the remaining specimens were positive for HSV by culture and 6 were positive for Adenovirus, also by culture. No causative agent was identified in 17 cases. Each PCR-positive sample was confirmed by Southern blot hybridization. All four positive specimens were also positive when PCR was performed using biotinylated primers against *C. trachomatis* specific cryptic plasmid. *Chlamydia* culture using McCoy cell monolayers detected *Chlamydia* in only two of the four PCR positives and one of these was also positive using the Microtrak fluorescent antibody detection system. In another preliminary study, PCR products were further evaluated using a panel of DNA probes in a dot blot hybridization method to identify the serovar of the *Chlamydia* PCR product (Kimura et al. 1993).

Toxoplasma

PCR has been used to study *Toxoplasma* infections in brain and ocular tissues. Diagnosis of retinal lesions in toxoplasmosis generally relies on clinical characteristics and course of the infection and must be differentiated from other causes of posterior uveitis including HSV, CMV, VZV, syphilis, fungi, etc. Because of the broad range of organisms to be considered in the differential diagnosis, the availability of molecular diagnostics would be of value.

PCR in one study was adapted to evaluate paraffin-embedded sections from enucleated eyes with clinical evidence of *Toxoplasma* retinitis (Brezin et al. 1990). Primers were chosen to detect the B1 intron and the P30 major surface protein gene. The B1 gene primers detected *Toxoplasma* in two of four sections from an enucleated eye in which *Toxoplasma* cysts had been documented histologically. The same primers also detected *Toxoplasma* in one of four sections from an eye with clinically apparent *Toxoplasma* retinitis but no detectable cysts. The P30 gene primers did not detect *Toxoplasma* in any of the sections, and it was thought that this could be due to strain variation in this antigen.

Bacterial ribosomal DNA

An interesting application of PCR was reported in one study designed to detect 16s bacterial ribosomal DNA in vitreous specimens. A double-nested PCR technique was used to test vitreous samples from 20 cases of clinically diagnosed delayed postoperative endophthalmitis and 27 normal control eyes that did not have prior surgery. PCR was positive in 2 of the 27 control samples and in 14 of 20 delayed endophthalmitis samples, five of which were also culture positive. These findings suggest that PCR may be effective in detecting a bacterial cause in delayed postoperative endophthalmitis and would be especially useful when bacterial cultures are negative.

Because a variety of ocular specimens have been shown to be conducive to analysis by PCR, it is plausible that systems that have been reported for other tissues or fluids may be applied to ocular specimens as well. For example, ocular involvement in Lyme disease is usually a late manifestation and may occur several months to years following the initial diagnosis. Because of this interval, the ocular findings (conjunctivitis, iritis, choroiditis, numular and interstitial keratitis, ulcerative keratitis, ischemic optic neuropathy, retinal hemorrhages or exudative retinal detachment) may not be associated with *Borrelia* infection. Specimens from the eye have not been tested by PCR; however, PCR systems to detect *Borrelia* using several different primers have been successfully used to test plasma, buffy coat cells, urine, and cerebrospinal fluid. PCR may be especially useful in central nervous system manifestations of the disease where the antibody response in the cerebrospinal fluid generally lags behind the clinical symptoms.

REFERENCES

Biswas J, Mayr AJ, Martin WJ, Rao NA: Detection of human cytomegalovirus in ocular tissues by polymerase chain reaction and in situ hybridization. Graefe's Arch Clin Exp Ophthalmol 1993; 231:66–70.

Brezin AP, Eqwuagu CE, Burnier M Jr et al.: Identification of Toxoplasma gondii in paraffin-embedded sections by the polymerase chain reaction. Am J Ophthalmol 1990; 110:599–604.

Crouse CA, Pflugfelder SC, Periera I et al.: Detection of herpes viral genomes in normal and diseased corneal epithelium. Curr Eye Res 1990; 9:569–581.

Erlich HA, Gelfand D, Sninsky JJ: Recent advances in the polymerase chain reaction. Science 1991; 252:1643–1651.

Faloona F, Weiss S, Ferre F, Mallis K: Direct detection of HIV sequences in blood:high gain polymerase chain reaction. Abstract 1019. 6th International Conference on AIDS, 1990; San Francisco, CA.

Fox GM, Crouse CA, Chuang EL et al.: Detection of herpesvirus DNA in vitreous and aqueous specimens by polymerase chain reaction. Arch Ophthalmol 1991; 109: 266–271.

Innis MA, Gelfand DH, Sninsky JJ, White TJ: PCR protocols. A guide to methods and applications. San Diego: Academic Press, 1990.

Kaye SB, Lynas C, Patterson A et al.: Evidence for herpes simplex virus latency in the human cornea. Br J Ophthalmol 1991; 75:195–200.

Kimura T, Saito J, Ashizaway et al.: Detection and serovar determination of Chlamydia trachomatis by PCR and dot-blot hybridization. Invest Ophthalmol Vis Sci 1993; 845.

Lauer SA, Malter JS, Meier JR: Human papillomavirus type 18 in conjunctival intraepithelial neoplasia. Am J Ophthalmol 1990; 110:23–27.

Loche M, Mach B: Identification of HIV-infected seronegative individuals by a direct diagnostic test based on hybridization to amplified viral DNA. Lancet 1988; ii:418–421.

Longo MC, Berninger MS, Hartley JL: Use of uracil DNA glycosylase to control carry-over contamination in polymerase chain reactions. Gene 1990; 125–128.

McDonnell JM, McDonnell PJ, Sun YY: Human papillomavirus DNA in tissues and ocular surface swabs of patients with conjunctival epithelial neoplasia. Invest Ophthalmol Vis Sci 1992; 33:184–189.

Mitchell SM, Fox JD, Tedder R, Lightman S: The use of polymerase chain reaction in the diagnosis and management of patients with presumed viral retinitis. Abstract. Invest Ophthalmol Vis Sci 1993; 34:1056.

Mullis KB, Faloona F: Specific synthesis of DNA in vitro via a polymerase-catalyzed chain reaction. Meth Enzymol 1987; 155:335–350.

Noonan KE, Robinson IB: mRNA phenotyping by enzymatic amplification of randomly primed cDNA. Nucleic Acids Research 1988; 16:10366.

Odrich MG, Jakobiec FA, Lancaster WD et al.: A spectrum of bilateral squamous conjunctival tumors associated with human papillomavirus type 16. Ophthalmology 1991; 98:628–635.

Ou CY, Kwok S, Mitchell SW et al.: DNA amplification for direct detection of HIV-1 in DNA of peripheral blood mononuclear cells. Science 1988; 239:295–297.

Pflugfelder SC, Huang A, Crouse C: Epstein-Barr virus keratitis after a chemical facial peel. Am J Ophthalmol 1990a; 110:571–573.

Pflugfelder SC, Crouse C, Pereira I, Atherton S: Amplification of Epstein-Barr virus genomic sequences in blood cells, lacrimal glands, and tears from primary Sjögren's syndrome patients. Ophthalmology 1990b; 97:976–984.

Qavi HB, Green MT, SeGall GK et al.: Frequency of infections of corneas with HIV-1 and HHV-6. Current Eye Res 1991; 11:315–323.

Rogers MF, Ou CY, Rayfield M et al.: Use of the polymerase chain reaction for early detection of proviral sequences of human immunodeficiency virus in infants born to seropositive mothers. New Engl J Med 1989; 320:1649–1654.

Rogers BB, Alpert LC, Hine EAS, Buffone GJ: Analysis of DNA in fresh and fixed tissue by the polymerase chain reaction. Am J Pathol 1990; 136:541–548.

Rong BL, Pavan-Langston D, Weng QP et al.: Detection of herpes simplex virus thymidine kinase and latency-associated transcript gene sequences in human herpetic corneas by polymerase chain reaction amplification. Invest Ophthalmol Vis Sci 1991; 32:1808–1815.

Saiki RK, Gelfund DH, Stoffel S et al.: Primer-directed enzymatic amplification of DNA with a thermostable DNA polymerase. Science 1988; 239:487–491.

Saiki RK, Scharf S, Faloona F et al.: Enzymatic amplification of beta-globin genomic sequences and restriction site analysis for diagnosis of sickle cell anemia. Science 1985; 230:1350–1354.

Sambrook J, Fritsch EF, Maniatis T: Molecular Cloning. A laboratory manual. 2d Ed. Plainview, NY: Cold Spring Harbor Laboratory Press, 1989.

Talley AR, Garcia-Ferrer F, Laycock KA et al.: The use of polymerase chain reaction for the detection of chlamydial conjunctivitis. Am J Ophthalmol 1992; 114:685–692.

Laboratory Training: Equipment, Maintenance, and Infection Control

11

The following guidelines may be used for general equipment maintenance and microbiology training schedules. A procedure and record of this maintenance is required by most outside quality control surveillance groups. Infection control should be exercised, and policies are suggested.

Equipment Quality Control

1. General principle:
   A. All equipment used in microbiology must be clean and properly maintained.
   B. Refer to the equipment quality control charts. Perform cleaning, function verification, and preventative maintenance indicated on the quality control charts.
   C. Keep a manufacturer's instruction manual near or immediately adjacent to each piece of equipment. See following Ocular Microbiology Training Program (11.2).
   D. For equipment not listed below, do preventive maintenance and function checks as directed by the manufacturer's instruction manuals.
   E. Infection control and proper use of biohazard material and equipment should be documented, and procedure lists available in the work area.

154

11.1 QUALITY CONTROL SURVEILLANCE PROCEDURES OF COMMONLY USED MICROBIOLOGY EQUIPMENT:

Equipment	Procedure	Schedule	Tolerance limits
Refrigerators	Recording of temperature	Daily or continuous	2° to 8°C
Freezers	Recording of temperature	Daily or continuous	−8° to −20°C −60° to −80°C
Incubators	Recording of temperature	Daily or continuous	34° to 37°C
Incubators	Measuring of CO_2 content (use blood gas analyzer, Fyrite device, or CO_2 measuring device built into incubator)	Daily	5% to 10% (CO_2)
Water baths	Recording of temperature	Daily	±10°C of setting
Heating blocks	Recording of temperature	Daily	± 1°C of setting
Autoclaves	Test with spore strip	At least weekly	No growth of spores (*Bacillus stearothermophilus*) in subculture indicates sterility
Anaerobic jars	Methylene blue indicator	With each use	conversion of strip from blue to white indicates low O_2 tension
Centrifuges	Check revolutions with tachometer	Monthly	Within 5% of dial indicator setting
Biologic safety hoods	Measure air velocity	Semiannually or quarterly	50 ft of air flow per min ± 5 ft/min

Note: Each monitoring thermometer must be calibrated against a standard thermometer.

Equipment Malfunctions, Unacceptable Results

A. If equipment malfunctions or if the tolerance limits on the quality control charts are exceeded, perform the obvious corrective step (e.g., adjusting incubator thermostat) and document in a Equipment Adjustment Log to be kept in the department.

B. If the problem cannot be corrected by laboratory personnel, depending on the equipment involved, do one or more of the following:

   1. Call the Maintenance Department.

2. Contact an authorized repair person.
3. Obtain parts recommended by manufacturer or repair station needed to correct the problem.
4. Replace the equipment.
C. Document all corrective actions, including replacement, in the Equipment Adjustment Record.

BIBLIOGRAPHY

Baron EJ: Instrument maintenance and quality control. Section 12. In Isenberg HD et al. (eds.): Clinical microbiology procedures handbook. Washington, DC: American Society for Microbiology, 1992.

Koneman EW: Color atlas and textbook of diagnostic microbiology, 4th Edition. Philadelphia: J.B. Lippincott, 1992: 55.

11.2 MICROBIOLOGY TRAINING PROGRAM

The ocular microbiologist should be familiar with and well oriented to the protocol and procedures used in an ocular microbiology laboratory. The following checklist will provide guidelines for the training of new staff. A photocopy of this chart can be used in your laboratory and given to each new member with space provided for initialing when completed.

11.2.1 Microbiology Training Program Part 1

Ocular Microbiology Techs   Name_____

	Supervisor	Comments	Date
1. General Orientation to Microbiology			
a. Location of CO_2, regular and fungal incubators	___	___	___
b. Location of culture media	___	___	___
c. Location of office supplies	___	___	___
d. Location of tissue grinders	___	___	___
e. Location of stain supplies	___	___	___
f. Location of requisitions, etc.	___	___	___
g. Accession and log-in procedure	___	___	___
h. Review ocular microprocedure book	___	___	___
2. Gram Stains			
a. Source protocol	___	___	___
b. Staining procedure	___	___	___
c. Cellular morphology	___	___	___
d. Interpretation	___	___	___
e. Quality control	___	___	___
f. Reporting protocol	___	___	___
3. Giemsa Stains			
a. Source protocol	___	___	___

    b. Staining procedure   ____   ____   ____
    c. Cellular morphology   ____   ____   ____
    d. Interpretation   ____   ____   ____
    e. Quality control   ____   ____   ____
    f. Reporting protocol   ____   ____   ____

11.2.2 Microbiology Training Program Part 2

    4. Primary Inoculation
        a. Source protocol   ____   ____   ____
        b. Processing of cultures   ____   ____   ____
            1. All sterile sites
                corneas, vitreous)   ____   ____   ____
            2. Conjunctiva, lids,
                (lacrimal, etc.   ____   ____   ____
            3. All fungal   ____   ____   ____
            4. All mycobacterium   ____   ____   ____
            5. All tissue specimens   ____   ____   ____
            6. All anaerobic requests   ____   ____   ____
            7. *Acanthamoeba* isolation   ____   ____   ____
            8. Miscellaneous
                and special requests   ____   ____   ____
        c. Processing of cultures
            set up by physicians   ____   ____   ____
        d. Quality control   ____   ____   ____
    5. Antimicrobial Removal Device
        a. Procedure   ____   ____   ____
        b. Intended use and specimen source   ____   ____   ____
        c. Secondary inoculation
            and incubation   ____   ____   ____
    6. Culture Reading and Interpretation
        a. Colony count and quantitation   ____   ____   ____
        b. Colonial morphology   ____   ____   ____
        c. Gram-negative
            identification schemes   ____   ____   ____
        d. Gram-positive
            identification schemes   ____   ____   ____
        e. Nonsaccharolytic gram-negative
            identification (*Haemophilus,*
            Neisseria, Moraxella, etc.)   ____   ____   ____
        f. Secondary and selective
            media inoculation   ____   ____   ____
        g. Subcultures   ____   ____   ____
        h. Optochin, Bacitracin zone
            interpretation   ____   ____   ____
        i. Spot tests (Beta-lactamase,
            oxidase, etc.)   ____   ____   ____

Supervisor Comments Date

j. Sceptor or Vitek, etc.
    system identification   ____   ____   ____
k. API identification system   ____   ____   ____
7. Yeast and fungal identification
m. Actinomycetes and *Mycobacterium*   ____   ____   ____
n. *Acanthamoeba* workups   ____   ____   ____
o. Anaerobic identification   ____   ____   ____
p. Reporting protocol   ____   ____   ____
q. Critical reporting procedure   ____   ____   ____
r. Quality control recording   ____   ____   ____
s. Source and age of culture
    filing system   ____   ____   ____
t. Physicians queries and
    telephone requests   ____   ____   ____
u. Sending out reports
    and preliminaries   ____   ____   ____
v. Filing of final reports   ____   ____   ____

11.2.3. Microbiology Training Program Part 3

8. Inventory, Ordering, and Checking Supplies
a. Storage requirements of reagents   ____   ____   ____
b. Checking of expiration dates   ____   ____   ____
c. Discard procedure for expired
    reagents   ____   ____   ____
d. Quality checks and control   ____   ____   ____
e. Location of reagents:
    Secptor, API, and spot test equipment
    Sensitivity disks
    All plated media   ____   ____   ____
f. Checking status of inventory levels   ____   ____   ____
g. Reporting and ordering procedure   ____   ____   ____
h. Temperature recording
    for refrigerators   ____   ____   ____

11.2.4. Microbiology Training Program Part 4

9. Familiarity with Ocular Involvement and Disease Processes
a. Anatomy of the eye   ____   ____   ____
b. Glossary of terms   ____   ____   ____
c. Laboratory diagnosis of
    corneal ulcers   ____   ____   ____
d. Clinical indications of ocular infection ____   ____   ____
e. Antibiotics of choice by source   ____   ____   ____
f. Infectious cycle of *Chlamydia*   ____   ____   ____
g. Endophthalmitis disease process   ____   ____   ____
h. Fungal keratitis and diagnosis   ____   ____   ____

11.3. LABORATORY SAFETY AND INFECTION CONTROL

11.3.1. Prevention of Laboratory-acquired Infection

Purpose
Because of the frequent contact between laboratory personnel and infectious materials, infection control within the microbiology laboratory is an important aspect of hospital infection control. **All** visitors and new laboratory personnel should be familiarized with the hazards of disease transmission within the laboratory.

Common causes of laboratory-acquired infections

Hepatitis and AIDS virus   A particular problem with glassware washing and those who come in contact with blood, semen, urine, and ocular fluids.

Tuberculosis   A problem when isolation of this causative agent is attempted or by contact with possible mycobacterium contaminated material, especially sputum.

Brucellosis   Infectious hazard when isolation of this pathogen is attempted or by contact with contaminated material, blood, ocular fluids, etc.

Shigella, Salmonella, Coccidioides, Neisseria meningitidis, *Amoebae, Q fever, etc.*   Although infrequently encountered, they are infectious enough to be considered among common causes of laboratory-acquired infections.

Common hazards

Accidents involving needles, syringes, broken glassware: **Cause:** Accidental puncture of skin with contaminated needles or infectious aerosols created when syringes are used improperly.

1. When a needle is being withdrawn through the stopper of a culture or vaccine bottle, an alcohol-soaked cotton ball should be used to shield the needle.
2. Clotted blood or pus should not be homogenized through a needle and only Luer-Lok syringes should be used in the laboratory.
3. All needles, glassware, and used syringes must be disposed of in biohazard containers kept in the laboratory for this purpose so as not to become a potential hazard to laboratory workers and other hospital personnel. Biohazard containers are double bagged and disposed of by incineration.

Diseases transmitted by mouth-pipetting or eating, drinking, or smoking in the laboratory   **Cause:** Pipets may become contaminated by contact with infectious material, and infectious aerosols can be created when the contents of a pipet are forcibly expelled. Food and drinks may become contaminated by infectious material and may provide a source of nutrition for infectious agents when left in the laboratory area or discarded into nonbiohazard containers. These are the most frequent preventable causes of laboratory acquired infections. In-depth procedures and preventative measures to protect laboratory workers and other hospital personnel should be contained in the general laboratory policy and procedures.

Surveillance of nosocomial infections

Laboratory results are a potential "early-warning system" for the emergence of highly infectious pathogens, multiply resistant organisms, and clusters of unusual infections.

1. Rapid dissemination of data from microbiologist to clinician may be facilitated by providing both preliminary and final copies of culture results.
2. A copy of positive results should be sent also to the infection control nurse to facilitate surveillance of infections requiring isolation or notification of public health authorities.

Regular assessment of specimen collection and handling may prevent inaccurate results caused by improperly collected or transported specimens. Ophthalmologists and microbiology personnel should be made aware of the protocol for collection and processing of ocular specimens for culture.

Recognition and evaluation of hospital-acquired infections depends on accurate and consistent identification of microorganisms and correct interpretation of culture results. Incomplete or misidentification of organisms may obscure real problems and make retrospective epidemiologic investigation impossible.

Laboratory records should be retained at least 2 to 3 years and culture data should be recorded so that results are readily available by type of specimen, pathogen, and date.

Both clinician and microbiologist should be aware of erroneous microbiology results related to inadvertent use of faulty or contaminated materials. Contaminated culture tubes, media, syringes, skin antiseptics, and penicillinase have all been implicated in outbreaks of "pseudobacteremia." Such sources of error must be considered when culture or stain results do not appear to reflect clinical or epidemiologic findings accurately.

Epidemiologically important or unusual isolates should be forwarded to state or local reference laboratories for special typing or identification procedures.

The health of laboratory personnel should be monitored routinely to assess the adequacy of infection control within the laboratory:

1. Staff should be given preemployment and annual skin tests for tuberculosis, followed by chest X-rays when indicated.
2. A record of laboratory accidents and their outcomes should be kept and work habits discussed with accident-prone individuals.
3. The possibility of laboratory-acquired disease should be considered whenever personnel develop unusual or infective illness.
4. Periodic screening of personnel for hepatitis-B seroconversion may be helpful in determining high-risk areas for hepatitis and acquired immune deficiency syndrome (AIDS) virus. The risk of acquiring the human immunodeficiency virus (HIV) led to a series of recommendations by the Centers for Disease Control (CDC) beginning in 1982. Universal precautions

were introduced in 1987, and these were expanded to include bloodborne pathogens in 1988. At least twenty-five cases of HIV infection of laboratory workers were summarized in the Occupational Safety and Health Administration in the United States. This prompted standards to be enacted requiring an employer of persons whose duties may result in exposure to adopt a written infection control plan to minimize or eliminate employee exposure. This includes barrier protection such as latex gloves, policies for handling needles, and adherence to good laboratory and housekeeping practices.

BIBLIOGRAPHY

1. Balows A, Hausler WJ, Herrmann KL, et al.: Manual of clinical microbiology, 5th Edition. Washington, DC: American Society of Clinical Microbiology, 1991: 49–57.
2. Weinstein RA, Allison GF: The role of the microbiology laboratory in surveillance and control of nosocomial infections. Am Soc Clin Pathol 1978:69(2):130.

Media Preparation Procedures: Culture Media

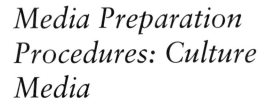

12

Microorganisms vary in their growth requirements. All organisms require sources of carbon, nitrogen, and trace elements. Some organisms use chemically simplified substances such as ammonia or nitrate, and others use free nitrogen. Certain organisms may require protein hydrolysates in the form of peptones, which can provide a more available form of nitrogenous compounds. These water-soluble peptones are derived from proteins by means of acid, alkali, or added enzymes. Most microorganisms have a limited ability to synthesize compounds alone and require complex compounds on which to grow. One should be aware of specific growth requirements in the preparation of media used for culture inoculation. The reader may wish to consult general microbiology textbooks for additional information concerning specific organisms such as Bergey's *Manual of Determinative Bacteriology* (1993).

Preparation
Dehydrated materials for media should be prepared in accordance with manufacturer's instructions. The use of chemically clean equipment and glassware is necessary to avoid contamination or trace chemical interference. Distilled or demineralized water of a neutral pH must be used unless otherwise specified. Dry materials must be carefully weighed, and water must be accurately measured. Solutions or ingredients requiring heat for sterilization of media may be performed by the use of direct heat, a boiling-water bath, or an autoclave and should be used for a limited time. Excessive heating may damage or carmelize media components.

pH of media and solutions

Microorganisms found in clinical ocular specimens grow best at a near-neutral pH; it is important to check the final pH of media prepared from dehydrated materials that have been opened or exposed to air, to detect any change that may have occurred.

Sterilization

1. Normal: sterilization is usually accomplished by autoclaving or by filtration. Volumes of up to 500 mL of most media are autoclaved at 121°C for 15 minutes. Larger volumes may need 20 to 30 minutes more.
2. Media containing carbohydrates: Temperatures from 116° to 188°C should be used for media containing heat-stable carbohydrates. The pH of these media should be checked before sterilization. For media containing heat-labile carbohydrates, the carbohydrates should be sterilized by filtration and added to cooled, autoclaved medium using aseptic techniques. Filters used to filter sterilize carbohydrates are available from Millipore (Bradford, MA). Carbohydrates also may be added by using impregnated paper disks. The dispensing of sterile media and the addition of sterile substances should be carried out in a laminar flow hood using strict aseptic technique (Nash and Krenz 1991).
3. Enriched media: Blood enrichments should be added aseptically to cooled base media, and avoid forming froth or bubbles during mixing. Media with blood enrichment must not be incubated before use. Sterility can be checked by placing several tubes or plates from each batch of medium in the incubator at 20° to 25°C or at 30° to 35°C for up to 7 days. The remainder must be refrigerated as soon as possible.

Quality control

Quality control of the media used is very important. The performance characteristics of biologic materials are determined by the nature of their origin and the methods of processing. There may be variations between lots or batches of ingredients. It is necessary to supplement or adjust media formulations to meet performance criteria. This can be accomplished with the use of American Type Culture Collection (ATCC) organisms and results should be recorded for each batch. Media that do not meet acceptable performance criteria cannot be used for patient specimens.

Sterility and media performance criteria

1. Materials used for preparation of media should indicate date of receipt, the manufacturer's instructions for storage, and expiration date.
2. Complete records should be kept for individual batches of medium prepared in your laboratory.
3. Approximately a 5% or 10% sample of individual batches of media require testing for sterility, particularly with those media to which various components are added after the basal media has been sterilized.
4. Records should include examination for color, clarity, and evidence of dehydration. Precipitates can occur in some media during storage. If these pre-

cipitates do not disappear on heating, the media must be discarded unless it normally contains some insoluble components.

5. The pH of each batch of medium is also checked electrometrically after completion or when medium base has cooled to room temperature. The pH should come into an acceptable range of ±0.2 of the value given by the manufacturer or package insert.

6. All media is then subjected to performance testing unless the reliability of a particular media has been ensured by extensive prior testing either within the laboratory or manufacturer. Within your laboratory, a collection of stock cultures with known typical culture characteristics adequate for testing all media used in the laboratory should be kept.

Manual performance testing

This is generally based on the use intended for the medium being tested and includes organisms that demonstrate both positive and negative reactions or growth. For multipurpose media, including blood agar plates, which may be used for the isolation of fastidious organisms and the demonstration of hemolysis, it is wise to use more than one test organism with variable expected reactions.

Media preparation

Many of these media are available from commercial sources. Be aware of the fact that different terminologies and spellings may be given, particularly with vendors from different countries. Do not hesitate to contact the manufacturers if questions arise; many of these have 800 numbers if calling from the United States. A FAX number is useful and should be obtained from vendors at the time of account setup.

Names and addresses of suppliers

1. BBL Microbiology Systems, Cockeysville, MD
2. Bristol Laboratories, Syracuse, NY
3. Burroughs-Wellcome Corporation, Research Triangle, Park, NC
4. Calbiochem-Behring, La Jolla, CA
5. Difco Laboratories, Detroit, MI
6. EM Science, Cherry Hill, NJ
7. Fisher Scientific CO., Pittsburg, PA
8. Flow Laboratories, McLean, VA
9. General Diagnostics, Anaheim, CA
10. ICN Pharmaceuticals, Inc., Cleveland, OH
11. Eli Lilly & Co., Indianapolis, IN
12. Merck & Co., Inc., Rahway, NJ
13. Marion Scientific Reagents, Kansas City, MO
14. Oxoid, U.S.A., Inc., Columbia, MD
15. Parke, Davis & Co., Detroit, MI
16. Pfanstiehl Laboratories, Nutley, NJ
17. Pfeizer Inc., New York, NY
18. Research Organics, Cleveland, OH
19. Roche Laboratories, Nutley, NJ

20. Sheffield Chemical, Union, NJ
21. Sigma Chemical Co., St Louis, MO
22. SYVA, Palo Alto, CA
23. E. R. Squibb & Sons, Princeton, NJ
24. The Upjohn Co., Kalamazoo, MI
25. Winthrop Laboratories, New York, NY

NOTE: There are a number of suppliers that carry these products or equivalent international brands. Check with the vendors for available suppliers in your country.

12.1 MEDIA PREPARATION PROCEDURES

12.1.1 Enriched Thioglycolate (THIO) Medium

Thioglycolate medium without indicator.. 30 g
Hemin (1% solution) .... 0.5 mL
Vitamin K_1 (1% solution) .... 0.1 mL
Distilled water .... 1 L

See Lombard-Dowell broth for directions to make 1% hemin and Vitamin K_1 solutions. Add all the ingredients; then heat to dissolve. Dispense 7 mL into 15-by 90-mm screw-capped tubes, autoclave at 121°C for 15 minutes, and cool. Place tubes in anaerobic jar, tighten caps, remove from anaerobic system, and store at 4°C or ambient temperature.

12.1.2. Enriched Thioglycolate Medium with 20% Bile (THIO + bile)

Prepare as described above, but add 20 g oxgall per liter of enriched thioglycolate medium before autoclaving (2% oxgall = 20% bile). Compare growth in bile medium with growth in enriched thioglycolate medium. You might want to use S for stimulated, N for no change, or I for inhibited when recording reactions.

12.1.3. Chopped Meat (CM) Medium for Anaerobes

Use BBL or DIFCO Manufacturer's prepared dry chopped meat or ground beef, lean (connective tissue trimmed off before putting meat through grinder)..
500 g
Distilled water .... 1 L
Sodium hydroxide (1 N solution)... 25 mL

Mix all ingredients, heat to boiling, then cool at 4°C overnight. Skim remaining fat from surface. Filter through several layers of gauze. Save the liquid filtrate. Wash the meat particles with distilled water two times to remove excess NaOH, and spread on a clean towel to partially dry. Add enough distilled water to the liquid filtrate to produce a final volume of 1 L.

Trypticase (BBL) .... 30.0 g
Yeast extract (DIFCO) .... 5.0 g
K$_2$HPO$_4$ .... 5.0 g
L-Cysteine .... 0.5 g
Hemin (1% solution) .... 0.5 mL
Vitamin K$_1$ (1% solution) .... 0.1 mL

See Lombard-Dowell broth for directions to make 1% hemin and Vitamin K$_1$ solutions. Mix all the ingredients listed, except for the L-Cysteine, heat to dissolve, and cool to 50°C. Add the L-Cysteine and mix to dissolve. Dispense 0.5 g meat into 15 × 90 mm screw-capped tubes. Add 7 mL enriched broth, autoclave at 121°C for only 15 minutes, and cool. Place tubes in anaerobic system, tighten caps, remove from anaerobe jar, and store at 4°C or ambient temperature. For record purposes, indication is made for chopped meat medium used to detect digestion (D) of meat particles, gas (G), or blackening (B) of the meat portion. Plain chopped meat broth is also an adequate holding medium for anaerobe stock cultures.

12.1.4. Thioglycolate Medium, Brewer Modified

Pancreatic digest of casein USP.. 17.5 g
Papaic digest of soybean meal USP.. 2.5 g
Glucose .... 10.0 g
Sodium chloride .... 5.0 g
Dipotassium phosphate .... 2.0 g
Sodium thioglycolate.. 1.0 g
Methylene blue... 0.002 g

Final pH 7.2 (may require adjustment). Dispense into test tubes, half full, and autoclave at 121°C for 15 minutes.

12.1.5. Thioglycolate Medium Without Indicator,* Plus Hemin

Pancreatic digest of casein USP.. 17.0 g
Papaic digest of soy meal USP .... 3.0 g
Glucose .... 6.0 g
Sodium chloride .... 2.5 g
Sodium thioglycolate... 0.5 g
Agar .... 0.7 g
L-Cysteine .... 0.25 g
Sodium sulfite .... 0.1 g
Purified water .... 1.0 L
Hemin .... 5.0 mg

1. Mix and heat with agitation to obtain solution.
2. Dispense into tubes with calcium carbonate chips or powder, approximately 0.1 g per tube, to promote viability, spore formation, and maintenance of cultures.
3. Boil and cool to room temperature just before use.
4. Add sodium bicarbonate that has been filter sterilized to a concentration of 1 g/mL and vitamin K_1 to a concentration of 0.1 g/mL.
5. Other supplements may be added, if desired, by introducing a pipet to the bottom of the tube and withdrawing the pipet as the supplement is added, for example, 5% Fildes enrichment or 10% sterile animal serum. Do not shake or invert tubes.

12.1.6. Thioglycolate Medium, Supplemented

Use thioglycolate medium without indicator prepared according to the manufacturer's insert instructions. Add hemin (5 µg/mL) and vitamin K_1 (0.1 µg/mL). Dispense into tubes, each containing a marble chip (Fisher); fill the tubes two-thirds to three-fourths full. Autoclave as directed. Just before use, boil or steam for 5 minutes, cool, and supplement with normal rabbit or horse serum (10% vol/vol) or peptic digest of sheep blood (Fildes enrichment [5% vol/vol]).

12.1.7. 5% Sheeps Blood Agar

Blood agar base
Brain heart infusion agar
Beef heart muscle, infusion from .... 375.0 g
Tryptose or Thiotone peptic digest of animal tissue USP .... 10.0 g
Sodium chloride .... 5.0 g
Agar .... 15.0 g
Distilled or demineralized water .... 1 L

Adjust to final pH 7.4. Autoclave at 121°C for 15 minutes. Cool to 50°C, and add 5% sterile defibrinated rabbit blood, if desired. For aerobic actinomycetes, add defibrinated horse blood, 50 mL/900 mL of base.

   Note: Blood or serum used for enrichment or in hemolysis determination should be from animals that are guaranteed free of antimicrobial agents. Defibrinated sheep blood is the blood of choice for routine work because the hemolytic reactions of streptococci on sheep blood are considered "true" and the growth of *Haemophilus haemolyticus*, which is often mistaken for hemolytic streptococci, is inhibited.

12.1.8. Other Blood-Enriched Products

Blood from other animal species, including humans, is often used to demonstrate hemolysis. However, hemolytic reactions on these bloods may be different from those observed with sheep blood, as follows:

1. Hemolytic reactions on defibrinated rabbit blood correlate with those of sheep blood; however, both *Haemophilus haemolyticus* and *H. influenzae* will grow on media containing rabbit blood.
2. Hemolytic reactions on defibrinated horse blood are not dependable, and some streptococci, for example, group D, demonstrate hemolytic reactions similar to those of group A.

   Note: It is not generally advisable to use blood from the blood bank because this blood contains citrates and glucose. Citrates are inhibitory to some organisms, and glucose may cause alpha- rather than beta-hemolysis. Antibodies and antimicrobial agents in human blood are known to cause inhibition of growth or false hemolytic reactions and sometimes both.

12.1.9. Chocolate Agars

Any one of the following could be used as required to obtain satisfactory growth with added components.

Beef infusion agar
Blood agar base
Casein peptone agar
Eugonic agar
Mueller-Hinton agar

Alternatively, GC Agar Base or GC Medium Base may be used.

Agar	10.0 g
Cornstarch	1.0 g
Pancreatic digest of casein USP	7.5 g
Peptic digest of animal tissue USP	7.5 g
(or substitute with another peptone using 15.0 g)	
Dipotassium phosphate	4.0 g
Monopotassium phosphate	1.0 g
Sodium chloride	5.0 g
Distilled water	1.0 L

Prepare sterile base medium. Add sterile 5% to 10% defibrinated blood, and heat at approximately 80°C for 15 minutes or until a chocolate brown color is observed.

Other variations of media

1. A chemical supplement such as 1% IsoVitalex (BBL) or Chocolate II (also BBL). These additives are described in the procedure for Thayer-Martin agar.
2. Yeast supplements may be added.
3. A double-strength medium may be prepared with addition of an equal volume of sterile 2% hemoglobin.
4. Chemical supplements may be added, particularly for *Neisseria* and *Haemophilus spp* isolation.

12.1.10. Thayer-Martin Agar

Combine sterile solutions, with the agar base cooled to 50°C. GC agar base sterile, double strength, 100 mL (see chocolate agars described previously). Add 2 g agar and 0.5 g glucose to the double-strength GC agar base before dissolving in 100 mL water.

Hemoglobin, 2% aqueous, 100 mL, or chocolated (heated) 5% defibrinated blood. Antibiotic inhibitors are added to give final concentrations per 100 mL medium of: vancomycin, 300 µg, colistin, 750 µg, nystatin, 1,250 U; trimethoprim lactate, 500 µg. Chemical enrichment, for example, 1% IsoVitaleX (BBL).

Vitamin B_{12} .... 0.01 g
L-Glutamine .... 10.0 g
Adenine .... 1.0 g
Guanine hydrochloride .... 0.03 g
P-Aminobenzoic acid .... 0.013 g
L-Cysteine .... 1.1 g
Glucose .... 100.0 g
Diphosphopyridine nucleotide oxidized (coenzyme 1) .... 0.25 g
Cocarboxylase .... 0.1 g
Ferric nitrate .... 0.02 g
Thiamine hydrochloride .... 3 mg
Cysteine hydrochloride... 25.9 g
Distilled water .... 1.0 L

Other supplements, such as supplement B11, may be used instead of the chemical enrichment described. For Martin-Lewis agar, use 400 µg vancomycin per 100 mL medium, and 200 µg anisomycin may be substituted for nystatin. For modified Thayer-Martin agar, add 2 g agar and 0.5 g glucose to the double-strength GC agar base before dissolving in 100 mL water.

12.1.11. Brain Heart Infusion Agar

General use for primary recovery of fungi from clinical specimens and may be used for ocular scrapings along with Sabauroud's dextrose agar

Agar .... 15.0 g
Protease or Gelysate (BBL) pancreatic digest of gelatin .... 10.0 g
Glucose .... 2.0 g
Sodium chloride .... 5.0 g
Disodium phosphate .... 2.5 g
Calf brains, infusion from .... 200.0 g
Beef heart, infusion from.. 250.0 g
Distilled or deionized water .... 1 L

Adjust to a final pH 7.4. Dispense and autoclave at 121°C for not more than 15 minutes. The use of freshly poured plates is recommended for isolation of *Actinomyces spp.*

12.1.12. Brucella Agar (Bacto Dehydrated)

Agar	15.0 g
Glucose or dextrose	1.0 g
Pancreatic digest of casein USP	10.0 g
Peptic digest of animal tissue USP (or peptamin)	10.0 g
Yeast extract	2.0 g
Sodium chloride	5.0 g
Sodium bisulfite	0.1g
Distilled water	1 L

Final pH 7.0 ± 0.2. 1 pound dehydrated medium (DIFCO) makes 16.2 L medium. Rehydrate with 28 g/L. Heat with agitation until dissolved. Dispense and autoclave at 121°C for 15 minutes. Cool to 50°C. Additives may be used for anaerobes.

For nonselective media:
1. Supplement before autoclaving with hemin (5 μg/mL), then, after autoclaving, with 50 mL sterile defibrinated sheep blood and 1 mL vitamin K_1 solution per liter.
2. Use 50 mL laked blood and 1 mL vitamin K_1 per liter. Prepare and use vitamin K_1 solution as follows:
   a. Weigh 0.2 g on a previously flamed aluminum foil square.
   b. Aseptically place 20 mL absolute ethanol in a sterile tube.
   c. Add foil, using a sterile forceps.
   d. When solution has occurred, remove foil. Final concentration is then 0.01 g/mL.
   e. Use 1 mL/L in agar media (concentration, 10 μg/mL).
   f. For fluid media, dilute stock solution 1:100 in sterile water. Use 0.01 mL/L (concentration, 0.1 μg/mL). Prepare and use hemin solution as follows:
   1) Dissolve 0.5 g hemin in 10 mL commercial ammonia water (or 1 N NaOH).
   2) Bring the volume to 100 mL with distilled water.
   3) Autoclave at 121°C for 15 minutes. Stock solution is 5 mg/mL. Use as a medium supplement with a final concentration of 5 μg/mL.

For Selective Media:
1. For *Bacteroides spp*, add kanamycin, 100 μg/mL, to brucella agar before autoclaving. Cool, and add blood and vitamin K_1 solution. Also add filter (0.45-μg pore size)-sterilized aqueous vancomycin to a final concentration of 7.5 μg/mL.

2. For *B. melaninogenicus*, add kanamycin as for other *Bacteroides spp*, first lysing the blood by freezing and thawing.

3. For *Clostridium spp*, and anaerobic cocci, add neomycin (110 μg/mL) before autoclaving. Add blood and vitamin K_1 just before pouring plates.

4. For certain *Fusobacterium, Eubacterium,* and *Clostridium* species, rifampin (50 μg/mL) and blood should be added just before pouring plates.

5. For *Fusobacterium* and *Veillonella* species, add neomycin (100 μg/mL) before autoclaving, add blood, vitamin K_1, and 7.5 μg vancomycin per milliliter before pouring plates.

12.1.13. Mueller-Hinton Agar

Agar .... 17.0 g
Beef infusion, from .... 300.0 g
Acid hydrolysate of casein .... 17.5 g
Starch .... 1.5 g
Distilled water .... 1.0 liter
Dispense, and autoclave at 116° to 121°C for 15 minutes. Cool to 45° to 50°C prior to addition of blood for sensitivity testing of *Streptococcus* spp and others.

12.1.14. Lowenstein-Jensen Medium

Monopotassium phosphate, anhydrous .... 2.4 g
Magnesium sulfate 7 H_2O .... 0.24 g
Magnesium citrate... 0.6 g
Asparagine .... 3.6 g
Potato flour.. 30.0 g
Glycerol .... 12.0 g
Distilled water .... 600.0 mL
Homogenized whole eggs.. 1 L
Malachite green 2% aqueous... 20.00 mL

1. Dissolve the salts and asparagine in the water.
2. Admix the glycerol and potato flour, then autoclave at 121°C for only 30 minutes. Cool to room temperature before addition of egg.
3. Use only eggs not more than 1 week old, scrub using 5% soap solution, then rinse thoroughly in cold running tap water.
4. Immerse in 70% ethyl alcohol for 15 minutes.
5. Break eggs into a sterile flask. Homogenize by hand shaking, then filter through approximately four layers of sterile gauze.
6. Add 1 liter homogenized eggs to the potato–salt mixture.
7. Prepare the malachite green and admix thoroughly.
8. Dispense 6 to 8 mL into 20-by-150-mm screw-capped tubes.
9. Slant, and coagulate in an inspissator or water bath or autoclave at 80°-85°C for 45 to 50 minutes.

10. Incubate for 48 hours at 37°C to check sterility, then keep stored at 4° to 6°C with caps tightly closed.

12.1.15. Middlebrook and Cohn 7H10, 7H11 Agars

7HIO agar. Stock solutions.
Solution 1. Store at room temperature.
Monopotassium phosphate .... 15 g
Disodium phosphate .... 15 g
Distilled water .... 250 mL
Solution 2. Store at 4° to 10°C.
Ammonium sulfate.. 5.0 g
Monosodium glutamate .... 5.0 g
Sodium citrate · 2H$_2$O USP.. 4.0 g
Ferric ammonium citrate... 0.4 g
Magnesium sulfate (7H$_2$O) ACS .... 0.5 g
Biotin, in 2 ml 10% NH$_4$OH .... 5.0 mg
Distilled water, to .... 250.0 mL
Solution 3. Store at 4° to 10°C.
Calcium chloride · 2H$_2$O ACS .... 50 mg
Zinc sulfate · 7 H$_2$O ACS .... 100 mg
Copper sulfate · 5H$_2$O ACS .... 100 mg
Pyridoxine hydrochloride.. 100 mg
Distilled water, to level... 100 mL
Solution 4. Clycerol reagent
Solution 5. Malachite green, 0.01% aqueous

Preparation procedure
1. To 975 mL distilled water, add
Solution 1 .... 25 mL
Solution 2 .... 25 mL
Solution 3 .... 1 mL
Solution 4 .... 5 mL
2. Adjust the final pH to 6.6 by adding approximately 0.5 mL 0.6 N HCL.
3. Add 2.5 mL solution 5 and 15 g agar.
4. Autoclave at 121°C for 15 minutes. Cool to 50° to 55°C, then add 100 mL OADC Enrichment:
Bovine albumin fraction V.. 5 g
Sterile saline, 0.85% .... 900 mL
Dissolve and add 30 mL of the following:
Oleic acid.. 0.6 mL
Distilled water, to .... 30.0 mL
Sodium hydroxide, 6 M .... 0.6 mL
Warm to approximately 56°C, and swirl until solution occurs.
5. Adjust to a final pH 7.0, measured electrometrically.
6. Add 40 mL sterile 50% aqueous glucose.
Sterilize by filtration.

7. Heat at 56°C for an additional hour, incubate overnight, heat again at 56°C, then once again incubate overnight at 37°C to check sterility.
8. Add 100 mL of this solution to agar base.
9. Also add 2 ml of membrane filter-sterilized freshly prepared catalase solution containing 1,000 µg/mL.
10. Dispense the complete medium into sterile petri plates or tubes.
11. Store at 4° to 8°C; unsealed and unprotected containers should not be used for longer than 4 to 7 days.
12. During preparation and storage, care should be taken to protect media from light.

7H11 agar
Add 1 g enzymatic casein hydrolysate per liter of 7H10 agar.

Selective 7H11 agar
Add the following antimicrobial agents per liter of 7H11 agar:

Carbenicillin	50 µg
Polymyxin B	200,000 U
Amphotericin B	10 µg
Trimethoprim lactate	20 µg

12.1.16. Sabouraud's Dextrose Agar

Agar	20 to 50 g
Glucose	40 g
Neopeptone or Polypeptone (BBL)	10 g
Pancreatic digest of casein USP)	5 g
Peptic digest of animal tissue USP	5 g
Distilled or deionized water	1 Liter

Adjust to final pH 5.6. Heat to dissolve completely. Dispense into tubes (18 to 25 mm in diameter), and autoclave at 121°C for 10 minutes.

Note: The addition of 10 mg thiamine per liter enhances the growth of some of the dermatophytes, especially *Trichophyton verrucosum*. If the dehydrated product is used or the medium is used for slide cultures, 2% agar should be used to insure a firm dry surface. The Emmons modification described in the following procedure is superior for most ocular fungal isolates.

Sabouraud's 2% dextrose agar (similar to Emmons)
For subculture of fungi to induce sporulation

Glucose	10 g
Bacto-Peptone (DIFCO)	
or Polypeptone (BBL)	10 g
or (Pancreatic digest of casein USP	5 g)
or (Peptic digest of animal tissue USP	5 g)

Agar .... 17 g
Distilled water .... 1 L
Adjust to final pH 6.9. Dispense and autoclave at 185° to 121°C for 10 minutes.

12.1.17. Sabouraud's Dextrose Agar (Emmons Modification)

Use   For the cultivation of fungi from ocular specimens.

The Emmons modification of Sabouraud's dextrose agar differs in that it has an approximately neutral pH and contains only 2% dextrose. A lower carbohydrate concentration has been found to be more conducive to growth and sporulation of common fungi found in ocular disease.

Sabouraud dextrose agar (Emmons modification)

Glucose .... 20 g
Bacto-Peptone or Polypeptone (BBL)................................... 10 g
(Pancreatic digest of casein USP .... 5 g)
(Peptic digest of animal tissue USP .... 5 g)
Agar .... 20 g
(or dried.. 17 g)
Distilled water .... 1 liter

Final pH 6.9 ± 0.1. Dispense, and autoclave at 118° to 121°C for 10 minutes.

Preparation
Suspend the dry ingredients in a liter of distilled water. Mix thoroughly to obtain a uniform suspension. Heat with frequent agitation and boil for 1 minute. Dispense and sterilize at 118° to 121°C (not over 15 lbs. pressure) for 15 minutes. Avoid undue exposure to heat, which encourages hydrolysis of the components and a consequent soft condition of the medium.

Use   It is used in the conventional manner for cultivation of fungi and recommended for all ocular specimens.

USP pancreatic digest of casein and USP peptic digest of animal tissue
Note: This media can be obtained in dehydrated form from BBL or DIFCO.

BIBLIOGRAPHY

Emmons CW, Binford CH, Utz JP: Medical mycology 3rd ed. Philadelphia: Lee and Febiger, 77.

12.1.18. Czapek Agar

Use   Recommended for species identification of aspergilli common in fungal keratitis and endophthalmitis in most parts of the world.

Agar .... 15.0 g
Czapek Dox medium
Sucrose .... 30.0 g
Sodium nitrate.. 3.0 g
Dipotassium phosphate .... 1.0 g
Magnesium sulfate .... 0.5 g
Potassium chloride .... 0.5 g
Ferrous sulfate.. 0.01 g
Deionized or distilled water .... 1 L

Adjust to final pH 7.3. Suspend 50 g of dehydrated material in a liter of distilled water. Mix thoroughly. When a uniform mixture has been obtained, heat with frequent agitation and boil for about 1 minute to dissolve the agar. Sterilize by autoclaving at 121°C for 15 minutes. Aseptically dispense into plates before the agar turns solid.

12.1.19. Potato Dextrose Agar

Useful for inducing spore production. Also commercially available from various manufacturers

Agar .... 15 g (or 20 g)
Peeled, diced potatoes, infusion from .... 200 g
Glucose .... 20 g
Deionized or distilled water .... 1 L

Procedure
Preparation as for other agar after infusion is made. The use of 2% agar provides a drier surface on the agar medium. Also available: Bacto Potato Dextrose dehydrated agar from Difco. 1 pound will provide 11.3 L medium. Suspend 39 g in 1 L of distilled or deionized water and heat to boiling dissolving completely. Sterilize in autoclave for 15 minutes at 15 lbs pressure at 121°C. Cool medium to 45° to 50°C and dispense into sterile petri dishes.

REFERENCES

Beneke ES, Rogers AL: Medical Mycology Manual, 4th Edition. Minneapolis: Burgess Publishing. 1980:33.
Difco Manual: Dehydrated culture media and reagents for microbiology, 10th Edition. Detroit, MI: Difco Laboratories, 1984:690–691.

12.1.20. Casein-Yeast Extract-Glucose Agar (CYG Agar)

For agar dilution susceptibility tests with imidazole antifungal agents

Agar .... 20.0 g

Casein hydrolysate .... 5.0 g
Yeast extract .... 5.0 g
Glucose .... 5.0 g
Distilled water .... 1 L

Adjust to final pH 7.0 ± .2

1. Dissolve by heat to boiling.
2. Dispense, and autoclave at 121°C for 15 minutes.

Casein yeast extract glucose broth (CYG broth)
For susceptibility testing with imidazole antifungal agents

Casein hydrolystate .... 5.0 g
Yeast extract .... 5.0 g
Glucose .... 5.0 g
Distilled water .... 1 L

Adjust to final pH 7.0 ± .21

1. Heat to dissolve.
2. Dispense, then autoclave at 121°C for 15 minutes.

12.1.21. Nonnutrient Agar Plates

For the isolation and culture of pathogenic freeliving amoebae such as *Acanthamoeba* and *Naegleria spp*

Agar .... 1.5 g
Page amoeba saline .... 100 mL

Dissolve agar in the saline with heat, and sterilize at 15 lb/in² pressure at 121°C for 15 minutes. Cool to 60°C and aseptically pour into sterile petri dishes. Use 29 mL for 100- by 15-mm dishes or 5 mL for 16- by 15-mm dishes. After the agar gels, store the plates in canisters at 4° to 5°C (refrigeration). Plates may be kept in the refrigerator for about 3 months.

Prepare Page amoeba saline as follows:

Sodium chloride (NaCl) .... 120 mg
Magnesium sulfate (MgSO$_4$ · 7H$_2$O) .... 4 mg
Calcium chloride (CaCl 2 · 2H$_2$O) .... 4 mg
Disodium hydrogen phosphate (Na$_2$ HPO$_4$) .... 142 mg
Potassium dehydrogen phosphate (KH$_2$PO$_4$) .... 136 mg
Distilled water, to .... 1,000 mL

Dissolve dry chemicals in water, and sterilize by autoclaving at 15 psi for 15 minutes. The solution may be stored in the refrigerator for up to 6 months. For *Acanthamoeba* isolation: also see procedure in previous sections.

1. Add a large inoculum of fresh (12 to 24 hours old) *E. coli* organisms to approximately 3 mL sterile page amoeba saline.
2. Using a sterile pasteur pipet, overlay onto nonnutrient agar plate containing clinical specimen.

REFERENCE

Cohn EJ, Buchanan HW, Laughrea PA, et al.: Diagnosis and management of acanthamoeba keratitis. Am J Ophthalmol 1985;100:389–395.

12.1.22. Chlamydia Media for the Cell Culture Isolation of *Chlamydia trachomatis*

A. *Growth Medium*
   Eagle minimum essential medium in Earle
   salts (10×) .... 50 mL
   Fetal calf serum .... 50 mL
   L-Glutamine, 200 mm solution .... 5 mL
   Sterile distilled water, to.. 500 mL
   Adjust the pH to 7.4 with 7.5% sodium bicarbonate.
B. Isolation medium is prepared by combining:
   Growth medium (see above) with added:
   Glucose .... 0.594 mg/mL
   Vancomycin .... 50 µg/mL
   Gentamicin .... 10 µg/mL
   Amphotericin B... 2 µg/mL
   Cycloheximide .... 1 to 2 µg/mL
   This medium can alternatively be used as a collecting medium by doubling the concentrations of vancomycin and amphotericin B.
C. Sucrose phosphate transport medium (USP)
   Sucrose .... 68.46 g
   K_2HPO_4.. 2.088 g
   KH_2PO_4... 1.088 g
   Distilled water .... 1,000 ml
   Adjust the pH to 7.0 and then autoclave before addition of:
   Bovine serum, to 5%
   Streptomycin.. 50 µg/mL
   Vancomycin .... 100 µg/mL
   Nystatin.. 25 U/mL
D. Sucrose-phosphate-glutamate transport medium (SPG)
   Sucrose .... 75.0 g
   K_2HPO_4.. 0.52 g
   Na_2HPO_4.. 1.22 g
   Glutamic acid .... 0.72 g
   Distilled water, to.. 1 L
   Adjust the pH to 7.4 to 7.6 then autoclave before addition of antibiotics described above (USP).

12.1.23. Mannitol-Salt Agar USP

Agar .... 15.0 g
Mannitol .... 10.0 g
Beef extract .... 1.0 g
Peptone or polypeptone (BBL)... 10.0 g
Sodium chloride .... 75.0 g
Phenol red .... 0.025 g
Distilled water .... 1.0 L

Adjust to final pH 7.4. Heat to dissolve, and autoclave at 121°C for 15 minutes.

12.1.24. MacConkey Agar

Agar .... 13.5 g
Bacto-Peptone or Gelysate (BBL)... 17.0 g
Peptone: Protease or Polypeptone (BBL)............................... 3.0 g
Lactose.. 10.0 g
Bile salts .... 1.5 g
Sodium chloride .... 5.0 g
Neutral red.. 0.030 g
Bacto Brom Cresol Purple or Crystal violet .... 0.001 g
Distilled water .... 1 L

Adjust final pH 7.1.

12.1.25. CTA Medium

Cystine Trypticase agar medium (BBL)

Agar .... 3.5 g
Cystine .... 0.5 g
Pancreatic digest of casein USP... 20.0 g
Sodium chloride .... 5.0 g
Sodium sulfite .... 0.5 g
Phenol red .... 0.017 g
Distilled water .... 1 L

Adjust to final pH 7.3. Mix and heat with agitation until solution occurs. Dispense, and autoclave at 115° to 118°C for not more than 15 minutes. Filter-sterilize carbohydrates and add to make a final concentration of 1%.

12.1.26. Rapid Sugar Test for *Neisseria* Species

Introduction
Neisseria gonorrhoeae and *N. meningitidis* can be presumptively identified in the clinical laboratory by growth and colonial morphology on selective media,

cell morphology and appearance on Gram stain, and oxidase reaction. It may be confirmed, generally, by either the fluorescent-antibody test, agglutination tests, or by its reaction on various carbohydrate media. The rapid test is a time-saving modification of the standard procedure for determining carbohydrate fermentation of glucose, lactose, sucrose, maltose, and fructose. It was originally developed for the testing of *Neisseria* but has been shown to be useful for other organisms such as *Haemophilus spp*, group DF-2, and *Kingella denitrificans*. Sugar utilization is useful for ocular isolates and may be set up from initial culture growth.

Reagents

Buffer-salt solution

KH_2PO_4	0.01 g
K_2HPO_4	0.04 g
KCl	0.80 g
Phenol red (1% aqueous solution)	0.40 g
Distilled water	100 mL

Adjust the pH to 7.0, filter, and store at 4°C in a sterile, screw-capped bottle.

Carbohydrate solutions   Prepare as 20% stock solutions in distilled water or broth (peptone, 10 g; meat extract, 3 g; sodium chloride, 5 g; distilled water, 1.000 mL). Adjust the pH to 7.0 and filter sterilize the solutions.

Procedure
1. Place 0.1 mL of the buffer-salt solution into each of five 10- by 75-mm sterile tubes.
2. Add 1 drop of the appropriate carbohydrate solution to each labeled tube.
3. Inoculate each tube with 1 drop of a very heavy 18- to 24-hour culture suspension prepared in 0.35 mL buffer-salt solution. Alternatively, a loopful of the suspected organism may be added directly into a tube of the buffer-salt-carbohydrate solution.
4. Incubate the tubes in a 35° to 37°C water bath for 4 hours, and read at 30-minute intervals.
5. A positive test is indicated by a yellow color (acid formation).

12.1.27. Urea Test Broth Urea Solution

Yeast extract	0.10 g
Monopotassium phosphate	0.091 g
Disodium phosphate	0.095 g
Urea	20.0 g
Phenol red	0.01 g
Distilled water	1 L

Sterilize by passing through a Seitz filter, and dispense 3-mL amounts into tubes. Alternatively, basal medium may be prepared in 900 mL distilled water, and autoclave at 121°C for 15 minutes. After cooling, add 100 mL 20% filter-sterilized urea solution and dispense the medium into sterile tubes. Inoculate with three loopfuls (2-mm loop) from an agar slant culture, then shake to suspend the bacteria. Incubate in a water bath or heat block at 37°C, and read after 10 minutes, 60 minutes, and 2 hours.

12.1.28. Motility Medium

Useful in identifying characteristics in anaerobes

Agar .... 4.0 g
Motility medium (Difco) .... 16.0 g
Nutrient broth... 4.0 g
Sodium chloride .... 1.0 g
Distilled water .... 1 L

Final pH 7.2 ± 0.1. Heat to dissolve the above ingredients, adjust the pH, dispense 7 mL into 15- by 90-mm screw-capped tubes, autoclave at 121°C for 15 minutes, and cool to 45°C. Place tubes in glove box or anaerobic condition, tighten caps, remove from glove box, and store at 4°C or ambient temperature.

Motility test medium

For Enterobacteriaceae:
Agar .... 4.0 g
Beef extract .... 3.0 g
Peptone or Gelysate (BBL)... 10.0 g
Sodium chloride .... 5.0 g
Distilled water .... 1 L

Adjust to final pH 7.4 Dispense approximately 8 mL per tube and autoclave at 121°C for 15 minutes.

For nonfermenting gram-negative bacteria (particularly pseudomonads):
1. Method of Gilardi
   Agar .... 3.0 g
   Pancreatic digest of casein USP .... 10.0 g
   Yeast extract.. 3.0 g
   Sodium chloride... 5.0 g
   Distilled water.. 1 L

Adjust to final pH 7.2. Dispense 3.5 mL per 13- by 100-mm tube. Autoclave at 121°C for 15 minutes.

BIBLIOGRAPHY

Gilardi GL (ed.): Glucose non-fermenting gram negative bacteria in clinical microbiology. West Palm Beach, FL: CRC Press, 1978.

12.1.29. Oxidation-Fermentation (OF) Test Medium

OF basal medium is commercially available.

For **Corynebacterium, Enterobacteriaceae, Aeromonas, Pseudomonas,** *and nonfermenting gram-negative bacteria*

Agar	3.0 g
Peptone (pancreatic digest of casein)	2.0 g
Sodium chloride	5.0 g
Dipotassium phosphate	0.3 g
Bromothymol blue	0.03 g
Distilled water	1 L

Adjust to final pH 7.1.

1. Dispense 3 or 4 mL per 13- by 100-mm test tube. Autoclave at 121°C for 15 minutes.
2. Cool to approximately 45°C, then add 10% glucose solution in distilled water for a final concentration of 1% glucose. Other carbohydrates such as dextrose may be substituted for glucose, if desired.
3. Dispense aseptically. This medium aids in the differentiation of organisms that use carbohydrates oxidatively rather than fermentation of pseudomonads and members of the tribe Mimeae. It also aids in the identification of organisms that do not use glucose in either way (e.g., *Alcaligenes spp*). Inoculate (stab) lightly two tubes of medium from a young agar slant culture. Cover one of the tubes with a layer (about 5mm) of sterile melted petrolatum or sterile paraffin oil. Incubate at 37°C, and observe daily for 3 or 4 days. Acid formation only in the open tube indicates oxidative utilization of glucose. Acid formation in both the open and the sealed tubes is indicative of a fermentative reaction. Lack of acid production in either tube indicates that the organism does not utilize glucose by either method, oxidation or fermentation.

For non-fermenting gram-negative bacilli

Pancreatic digest of casein	0.2 g
Phenol red, 1.5% aqueous	0.2 g
Distilled water	100.0 mL

1. Warm to dissolve the peptone and adjust the pH to 7.3.
2. Dissolve 0.3 g of agar by heating.
3. Dispense 6 mL per 16 × 125-mm test tube. Autoclave at 121°C for 15 minutes.
4. When basal medium is melted, add Seitz-filtered carbohydrate (glucose, D-xylose, D-mannitol, lactose, sucrose, or maltose) aseptically to a final 1% concentration.

BIBLIOGRAPHY

Gilardi GL (ed.): Glucose non-fermenting gram negative bacteria, in Clinical microbiology. West Palm Beach, FL: CRC Press, 1978.

12.1.30. API Oxidation-Fermentation Glucose Medium

Introduction
API Oxidation-Fermentation (OF) is intended to enable laboratory personnel to differentiate oxidation from fermentation metabolism of glucose by gram-negative bacteria. It is designed to be used in conjunction with the API 20E to assist in the identification of non-*Enterobacteriaceae* gram-negative bacteria.

Chemical and physical principles
API OF consists of glucose medium. This medium is inoculated and incubated so that organisms react with the glucose and read when the indicator system is affected by the metabolites, generally after 18 to 24 hours' incubation at 35° to 37°C.

Reagents and materials
API OF glucose ampules
(Glucose, tryptone, sodium chloride, dipotassium phosphate, agar, bromthymol blue)
Test tube rack
Water bath
Burner
Inoculation loop or needle

Procedure
1. Storage
   API OF should be stored in an upright position at 2° to 8°C refrigerator until used.
2. Preparation of medium
   a. Before inoculation of API OF, it is recommended that the medium be liquefied in a boiling water bath. Remove the ampules from the water bath, place in an upright position, and allow them to cool to room temperature before use
   b. Record the patient's specimen number on two of the ampules.
3. Inoculation of the Ampules
   a. To open the ampule, snap the top off by applying thumb pressure at the base of the flattened end of the plastic cap and discard the glass top. Replace the cap.
   b. With a flamed inoculating loop or needle, carefully pick a well-isolated colony, at least 3 to 5 mm in diameter or several pinpoint colonies of some morphology.
   c. Remove the cap from the OF ampule and inoculate by stabbing to a depth of approximately 10 mm. Replace the plastic cap.
   d. Remove the cap from a second OF ampule. Without flaming the loop, inoculate the second OF ampule by stabbing to a depth of approximately 10 mm. Replace the plastic cap.
   e. After inoculation, overlay one of the ampules with approximately 1 mL mineral oil.
4. Incubation
   a. After inoculation, incubate the OF ampule in a 35° to 35°C incubator.

    b. Reading should be made after 24 hours. Negative tubes should be incubated for an additional 24 hours.

5. Reading of the Ampules

    a. After 24 hours of incubation, the reactions are read and recorded on the API 20E worksheet. Oxidative utilization of glucose is indicated by the production of acid in the open (OF-O) tube only. With fermentative utilization, acid will be produced in both the open (OF-O) and overlayed (OF-F) ampules.

    b. All negative OF ampules should be reincubated for an additional 24 hours.

    c. Final readings should be made after 24 hours of incubation, when necessary.

    d. After all reactions have been recorded on the worksheet, the ampules should be autoclaved before disposal.

Interpretation

API OF	Positive	Negative
OF-O Oxidation (OF-O)	Any shade of yellow	Blue or no change
OF-F Fermentation	Yellow	Any shade of blue or no change

Note:

1. Oxidative organisms will produce acid in the OF-O ampule only.

2. Fermentative organisms will produce acid in both OF-O and OF-F ampules.

3. If the OF-F ampule is positive, the OF-O ampule must also be positive.

4. Lack of acid production in either tube indicates that the organism does not utilize glucose by either method.

Quality control

API OF has been quality controlled by standard testing procedures. Each lot is controlled with the stock cultures for sensitivity and specificity. For those who wish to do their own quality control, standard testing from the ATCC, Rockville, Maryland, is recommended.

Cultures

1. *Klebsiella pneumoniae* ATCC 13883
2. *Pseudomonas aeruginosa* ATCC 10145
3. *Alcaligenes faecalis* ATCC 8750

BIBLIOGRAPHY

API Analytab Products, Division of Sherwood Medical, New York.

12.1.31. Lombard-Dowell (LD) Broth Medium for Anaerobes

Trypticase (BBL) .... 5.0 g
Yeast extract (Difco) .... 5.0 g
Sodium chloride .... 2.5 g
Sodium sulfite .... 0.1 g
L-Tryptophan.. 0.2 g
Hemin (1% solution) .... 1.0 mL
Vitamin K1 (I% solution) .... 1.0 mL
Agar .... 0.7 g
Distilled water 1/Liter

Dissolve the L-Tryptophan in 5 mL 1 N NaOH before combining with the other ingredients. For a stock solution of hemin, dissolve 1 g in 20 mL 1 N NaOH, and add distilled water to make a final volume of 100 mL. For a 1% stock solution of vitamin K, suspend 1 g in 99 mL absolute ethanol. Heat to dissolve the ingredients, and adjust the pH. Dispense 7 mL into 15- by 90-mm screw-capped tubes, autoclave at 121°C for 15 minutes, and cool. See note in CHO fermentation broth for anaerobes. Place tubes in anaerobic system, tighten caps, remove from anaerobe jar, and store at 40°C or ambient temperature.

BIBLIOGRAPHY

Difco manual. Detroit: Difco Laboratories Inc., 1984.

Holt JG, Krieg NR, Sneath PHA, et al. (eds.): Bergey's manual of determinative bacteriology, 9th Edition. Baltimore: Williams & Wilkins, 1993.

Koneman EW, Allen S, Dowell VR, Sommers HM: Color atlas of clinical microbiology. 4th Edition. Philadelphia: J.B Lippincott, 1992.

Nash P, Krenz MM: Culture Media. Chapter 121. In Balows A, Hausler WJ, Herrman KL, et al.: Manual of clinical microbiology, 5th Edition. Washington, DC: American Society for Microbiology, 1991:1226–1314.

Wicklund GD, Horton BK (eds.): Manual of product technical data sheets. Tualatin, OR: PML Microbiologicals, 1990.

Glossary

Allergy	A hypersensitivity state caused by exposure to a particular allergen. Usually produces marked crinkly lid edema of one or both eyes and may be caused by topical agents such as eyedrops, other drugs, cosmetics, or plant allergens.
Blepharitis	Inflammation of the lid margins with redness, thickening, and often the formation of scales and crusts or marginal ulcers.
Blepharodermatitis	Inflammation of the margin of the eyelid and adjacent tissue.
Canaliculitis	Inflammation of the tubular passage in the eyelid that connects the punctum to the lacrimal sac.
Cavernous sinus thrombosis	Thrombosis of the cavernous sinus usually results from direct spread of infection along the venous channels draining the orbit and face.
Cellulitis, orbital	Inflammation of the orbital tissues resulting from infection that extends from the nasal sinuses or teeth, by metastatic spread of infection elsewhere, or from introduction of bacteria caused by orbital trauma.
Cellulitis, preseptal	Inflammation of the subcutaneous tissue of the eyelids; contained in the spaces defined by the fibrous attachments of the skin to the superior and inferior orbital rims and posteriorly by the orbital septum.

Chalazion	Chronic granulomatous enlargement of a meibomian gland caused by occlusion of its duct.
Chemosis	Edema of the conjunctiva.
Conjunctivitis	Inflammation of the delicate membrane tissue lining the eyelids and eyeball connected to the sclera and corneal tissue.
Conjunctivitis, acute	An acute conjunctival inflammation caused by bacteria, viruses, or severe allergies.
Conjunctivitis, allergic (vernal)	A bilateral chronic conjunctivitis allergic in origin, often seasonal.
Conjunctivitis, chronic	A chronic inflammation of the conjunctiva characterized by exacerbations and remissions that occur over months or years.
Conjunctivitis, giant papillary	Inflammation of the superior tarsal conjunctiva characterized by hyperemia and hypertrophy.
Conjunctivitis, inclusion	An acute conjunctivitis caused by *Chlamydia trachomatis;* usually refers to the endemic, nonbinding form of conjunctivitis affecting children and adults in urban areas as opposed to the severe, endemic infection (see *trachoma*).
Conjunctivitis, neonatal (*Syn:* ophthalmia neonatorum)	Inflammation of the conjunctiva characterized by purulent ocular discharge during the first 4 weeks of life. Major causes are chemical, chlamydial, and bacterial.
Corneal ulcer	Local defect or excavation of the corneal tissue caused by invasion by microorganisms, trauma, or hypoxia.
Dacryoadenitis	Inflammation of the lacrimal gland.
Dacryocystitis	Infection of the lacrimal sac, often secondary to nasolacrimal duct obstruction.
Dacryostenosis	Stricture of the nasolacrimal duct, often as a result of an infection or congenital abnormality.
Endophthalmitis	Inflammation of the ocular cavities and intraocular tissues restricted to the uveal tract, vitreous body, and retina.
Epiphora	Overflow of tears caused by faulty drainage by the outflow structures.
Episcleritis	Inflammation of the episcleral tissues, usually localized.
Entropion	Inversion of the eyelid causing irritation as the lashes rub against the globe; may lead to corneal ulceration and scarring. A common sequelae of old trachoma infections.

Foreign bodies	Conjunctival and corneal injuries by foreign bodies are the most frequent eye injuries and may lead to secondary infection.
Herpes simplex keratitis	Corneal herpes simplex virus infection, characterized by a spectrum of clinical appearances commonly leading to chronic inflammation, vascularization, scarring, and loss of vision.
Hordeolum (syn: sty)	An acute localized pyogenic infection of one or more of the glands of Zeis or Moll or of the meibomian glands.
Hypopyon	Accumulation of inflammatory cells and exudate in the interior chamber, producing a fluid level macroscopically visible in the inferior portion.
Interstitial keratitis	A chronic nonulcerative infiltration of the deep layers of the cornea, with uveal inflammation.
Iridocyclitis	Inflammation of the iris and ciliary body.
Iritis	Inflammation of the iris.
Keratitis	Inflammation of the cornea.
Keratitis, punctate superficial	Inflammation of the superficial epithelium of the cornea characterized by irregular and elevated diseased cells or small discrete superficial opacities and staining areas.
Keratitis sicca	Keratoconjunctivitis sicca; caused by the reduction of aqueous component of the preocular tear film; characterized by dryness and hyperemia of the conjunctiva and corneal erosion.
Keratocentesis	Surgical puncture of the cornea to obtain intraocular fluid (aqueous).
Keratomalacia	Xerophthalmia; a condition associated with vitamin A deficiency and characterized by a hazy cornea and dry eye.
Keratomycosis	Fungal infection of the cornea.
Keratoplasty	Corneal grafting; transplantation of donor corneal material to replace scar tissue that interferes with vision.
Kermes	An insect found on the leaves of various oaks, chiefly on *Oercus coccifera,* which furnishes a red pigment. An old folk remedy that after long-term use causes cicatrization of the conjunctiva.
Lacrimal	Pertaining to the tears. The lacrimal gland apparatus is responsible for the secretion of tears and lysozyme.
Leber's cell (Theodor Leber, German ophthalmologist, 1840–1917)	A macrophage often found in the Giemsa-stained conjunctival scrapings of patients with active trachoma.

Macula	A moderately dense scar of the cornea that can be seen without special optical aids.
Mucormycosis, ocular	A mycosis, usually occurring as an orbital cellulitis, caused by fungi of the order Mucorales. It may occur as a complication of a chronic debilitating disease, particularly diabetes, in which spores germinate and mycelial growths metastasize to other organs; often fatal.
Panophthalmitis	Inflammation of all the structures and tissues of the eye and usually causing its complete destruction.
Phlyctenular keratoconjunctivitis	A conjunctivitis usually occurring in children, characterized by nodular areas of inflammation and resulting from the atopic reaction of a hypersensitive conjunctiva or cornea to an unknown allergen.
Proptosis	Forward displacement of the eyeball.
Retinitis	Inflammation of the retina.
Retinovitritis	Inflammation of the retina and area of the vitreous immediately in front of the retina.
Sympathetic ophthalmia	A severe bilateral granulomatous uveitis that occurs as a hypersensitivity reaction to uveal pigment after trauma to one eye.
Tear dysfunction state	An abnormal condition caused by alteration of one or more of the components of the preocular tear film.
Trachoma	A chronic conjunctivitis caused by *Chlamydia trachomatis* and characterized by progressive exacerbations and remissions with follicular subconjunctival hyperplasia, corneal vascularization, and cicatrization of the conjunctiva, cornea, and lids.
Uvea, uveal tract	The vascular middle coat of the eye composed of the iris, ciliary body, and choroid.
Uveitis	Inflammation of the uvea.
Uveitis, lens-induced	A type of inflammation of the uvea caused by dissolution of the lens.
Vitrectomy	Partial or total excision of the gel-like fluid within the vitreous cavity.
Vitritis	Inflammation within the vitreous cavity.

BIBLIOGRAPHY

Berkow R (ed.): The Merck manual of diagnosis and therapy, 14th Edition. Rahway, NJ: Merck Sharp & Dohme Research Laboratories, 1987:1976–2015.

Dorland's Illustrated Medical Dictionary, 26th Edition. Philadelphia: W.B. Saunders, 1985.

Jones DB, Liesegang TJ, Robinson NM: Laboratory diagnosis of ocular infections, Cumitech 13. American Society for Microbiology, Washington, DC: 1981:26.

Index

Page numbers in *italics* refer to figures or plates